W9-BJB-152

Dr. Ann's Eat Right for Life®

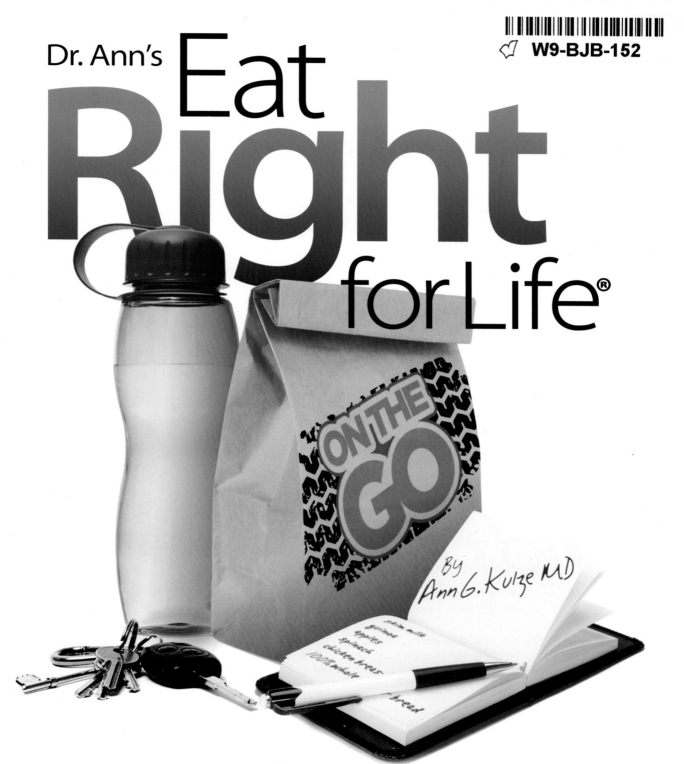

ON THE GO

By Ann G. Kulze MD

skim milk
quinoa
apples
spinach
chicken breast
100% whole
bread

Editorial Staff

Author: Ann G. Kulze, MD

Executive Editor: David Hunnicutt, PhD

Managing Editor: Brittanie Leffelman, MS

Contributing Editors: Madeline Jahn, MOL, Elizabeth Kulze, Carie Maguire

Creative Director: Brittany Stohl

Multimedia Designer: Adam Paige

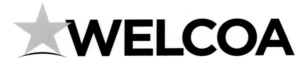

17002 Marcy Street, Suite 140 | Omaha, NE 68118
PH: 402-827-3590 | FX: 402-827-3594 | welcoa.org

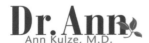

Ann Kulze, MD
CEO
78 Society Street
Charleston, SC 29401
PH: 843.329.1238
www.DrAnnwellness.com

Table of Contents

About **WELCOA**

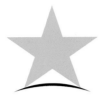

The Wellness Council of America (WELCOA) was established as a national not-for-profit organization in the mid 1980s through the efforts of a number of forward-thinking business and health leaders. Drawing on the vision originally set forth by William Kizer, Sr., Chairman Emeritus of Central States Indemnity, and WELCOA founding Directors that included Dr. Louis Sullivan, former Secretary of Health and Human Services, and Warren Buffet, Chairman of Berkshire Hathaway, WELCOA has helped influence the face of workplace wellness in the US.

Today, WELCOA has become one of the most respected resources for workplace wellness in America. With a membership in excess of 5,000 organizations, WELCOA is dedicated to improving the health and well-being of all working Americans. Located in America's heartland, WELCOA makes its national headquarters in one of America's healthiest business communities—Omaha, Nebraska.

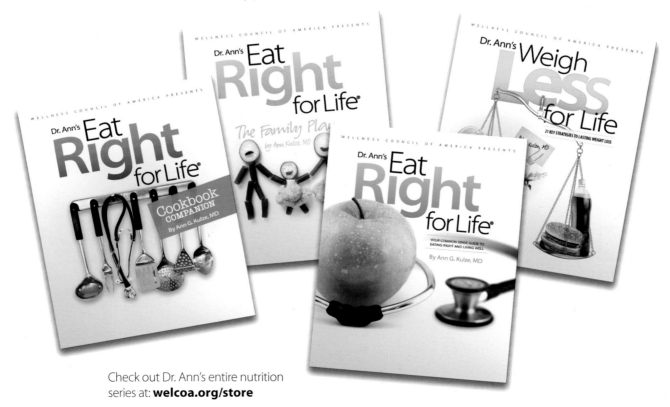

Check out Dr. Ann's entire nutrition series at: **welcoa.org/store**

About **Ann G. Kulze, MD**

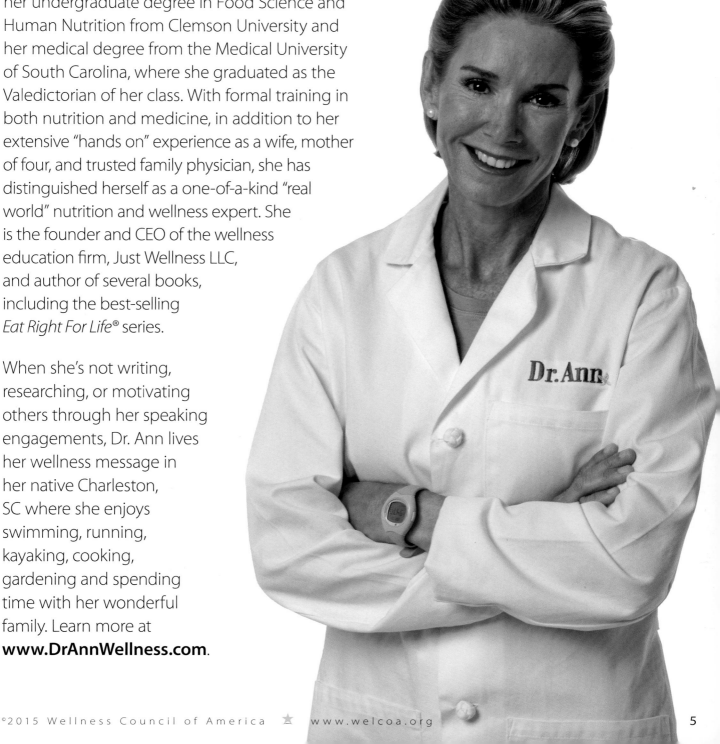

Ann G. Kulze, MD is a renowned authority on nutrition, healthy living, and disease prevention. She received her undergraduate degree in Food Science and Human Nutrition from Clemson University and her medical degree from the Medical University of South Carolina, where she graduated as the Valedictorian of her class. With formal training in both nutrition and medicine, in addition to her extensive "hands on" experience as a wife, mother of four, and trusted family physician, she has distinguished herself as a one-of-a-kind "real world" nutrition and wellness expert. She is the founder and CEO of the wellness education firm, Just Wellness LLC, and author of several books, including the best-selling *Eat Right For Life®* series.

When she's not writing, researching, or motivating others through her speaking engagements, Dr. Ann lives her wellness message in her native Charleston, SC where she enjoys swimming, running, kayaking, cooking, gardening and spending time with her wonderful family. Learn more at **www.DrAnnWellness.com**.

From
Dr. Hunnicutt

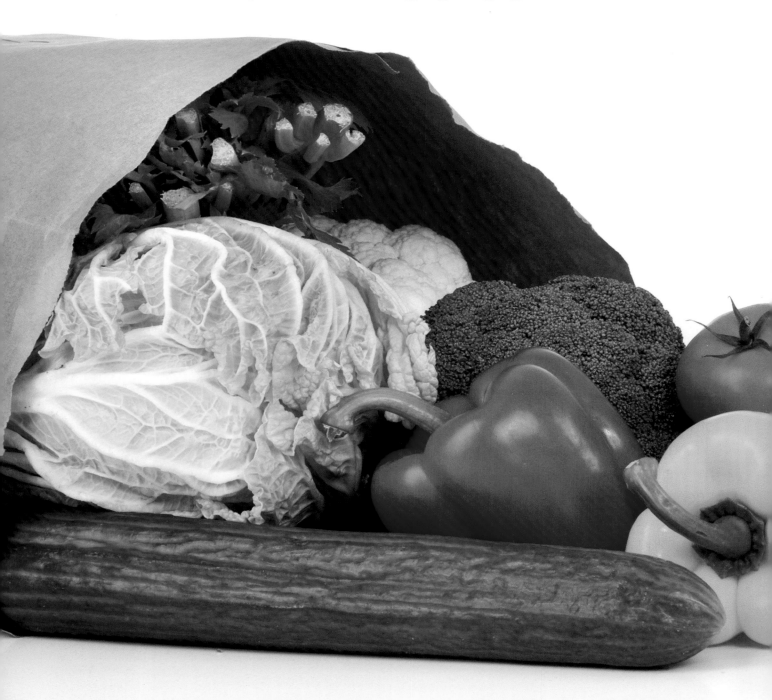

The third book in the trilogy of best-selling, nationally-acclaimed healthy eating guides authored by Dr. Ann Kulze, *Eat Right For Life®: On The Go*, should be considered essential reading for anyone interested in staying healthy in a fast food world.

In her first two books, Dr. Ann introduced the art and science of eating right for life and backed it up with a collection of smart, healthy and ridiculously delicious recipes. Now in her third book, she tackles the problem of how everyday people—folks like you and me—can exist (and indeed thrive) in a world that encourages us to eat most of our meals away from home.

In this book you will find information that is essential to staying healthy. Specifically, Dr. Ann will provide you with guidance on eating better in both fast food and higher-end restaurants. In addition, she'll offer up a mountain of sound advice in helping you eat better on the go.

As always, we are grateful to Dr. Ann for her wisdom and passion and her willingness to share both with people of all ages and from all walks of life. I have no doubt that you will find this book to be one of the most valuable books you've ever read.

Warmest Regards,

David Hunnicutt, PhD
President
Wellness Council of America

About Dr. David HUNNICUTT

Since his arrival at WELCOA in 1995, David Hunnicutt, PhD has developed countless publications that have been widely adopted in businesses and organizations throughout North America. Known for his ability to make complex issues easier to understand, David has a proven track-record of publishing health and wellness material that helps employees lead healthier lifestyles. David travels extensively advocating better health practices and radically different thinking in organizations of all kinds.

On The Go

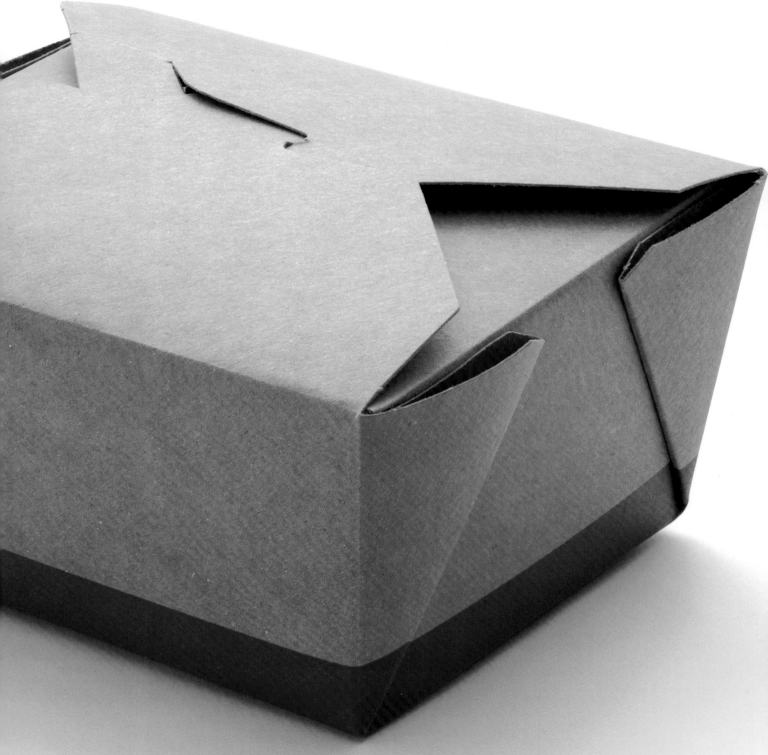

Being able to make the right food choices, no matter where you find yourself, offers an unrivaled opportunity to optimize your health and vitality. This book is devoted to this all-powerful singular goal. In the pages that follow, I am going to equip you with the real-world personal tools and knowledge required to healthfully navigate through our modern food landscapes. Whether you're in the grocery store, a fast food joint, or at the motel breakfast bar, I am going to make sure you have the information and guidance you need to select the foods that are best for you.

As a physician who has devoted her professional life to nutrition and wellness education, I know that the most challenging aspect of healthy eating is safely maneuvering through our food environments. Unfortunately, our modern food culture has become insanely toxic, and on virtually every single level. We currently produce enough food in this country to feed every man, woman, and child almost twice as many calories as they need. Even worse, most of what makes up this constant deluge of calories are processed, nutritionally defunct, manufactured foods—the very foods that dump even more disease-promoting agents like sodium, bad fats, sugar, and refined carbohydrates into an already noxious nutritional environment. Yes, bad-for-you foods are now super-accessible and everywhere. This tragic scenario is particularly perilous because our meal-time surroundings are the single greatest determinant of what and how much we eat. This single factor can trump self-control, hunger, knowledge, and even taste as the overriding determinate of what we consume, and most people are utterly unaware of this reality. Our food culture has undergone more negative changes in the last 40 years than in the previous 40,000, a fact that is unquestionably related to the dramatic uptick in the diet-related chronic diseases that now plague us. To put it straight—our food environments matter, and matter big time! This brings me right to the heart of the invaluable information contained in this book.

What you have in your hands is a harmonious and sustaining marriage between the best nutrition science, and three and a half decades of my personal experience as a healthy-eating aficionado—a wife, mother, nutrition expert, and working woman living and eating in the real world. Just like you—I grocery shop regularly for my family, dine out, eat at the office, get hungry in the convenience store, and have times when I'm forced to eat on the road. Despite the enormous pressures I experience to eat too much and to eat the wrong foods, I have enjoyed resounding success in maintaining nutritional excellence, a healthy body weight, and exceptional health. And now you can too! I wrote this book to share all of the tips, tactics, strategies, and rules that I know have been fundamental to my personal triumph. In these busy times, I promise you that my guidance will be straightforward, prescriptive, upfront, and comprehensive. I am determined to inspire and motivate you to become the master of your nutritional environment, and will make sure you know how to decipher the good from the bad. No matter the places and situations where you encounter food outside of your home, this book will take you straight to the choices that nourish and sustain you. Together we will take an aisle-by-aisle tour through the grocery store where I will tell you exactly what to buy and what to leave on the shelf. We will venture into the crazy world of dining out where you will learn how to leave with your health and body weight in check and a tasty and satisfying meal in your stomach. We will make a road trip through the airports and onto the highways where you will see that you can maintain your healthy regimen even while on the go. Lastly, we will tackle eating in the workplace so you can perform at the top of your game and still have plenty of energy left over for your loved ones.

With the wisdom that follows, I know you can confidently stand up to our big, scary food culture. I know you will succeed because by the end of this book you will understand how to rely on the right foods that are always ready and waiting as your indefatigable ally in the quest for radiant health. Although they are sorely outnumbered by the wrong foods, I promise there will be healthy choices by your side every step of the way. So let's roll!

—*Ann G. Kulze, MD*

Healthy Grocery Shopping

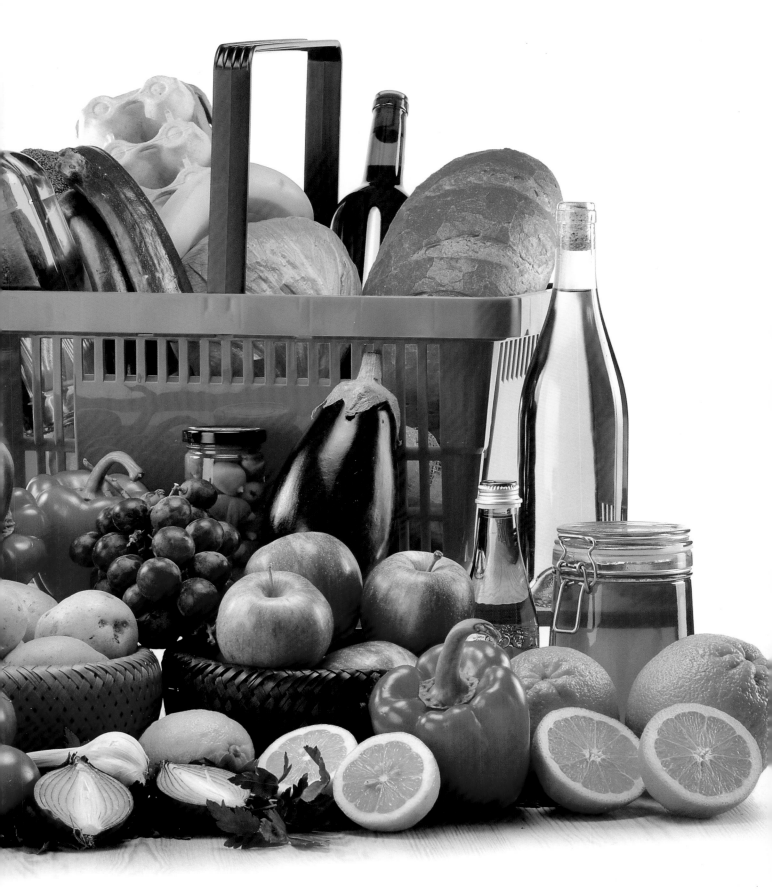

Healthy Grocery Shopping

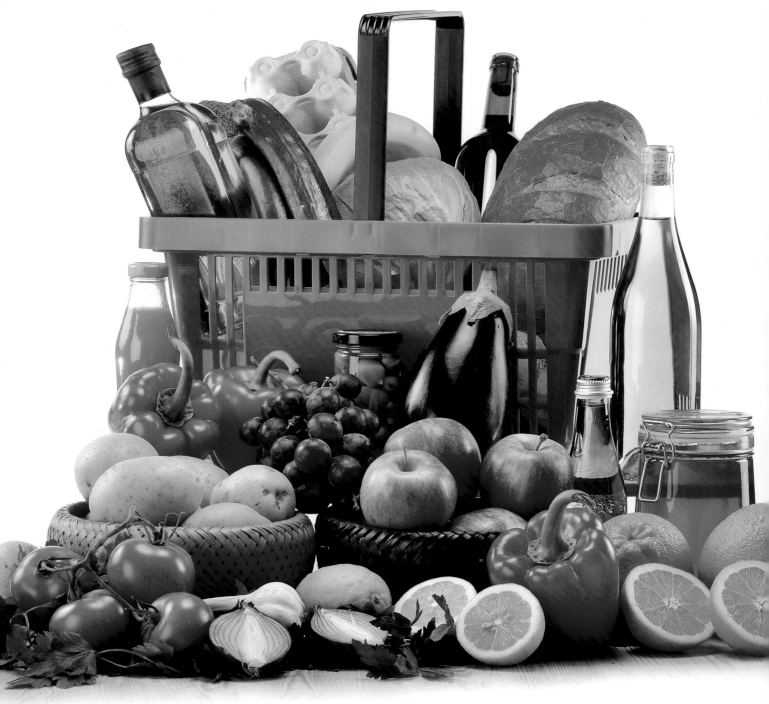

Healthy eating begins in the grocery store. Learning how to healthfully navigate through the supermarket aisles and select the right foods provides one of the most powerful opportunities to improve you and your family's health and well-being.** Today the science is now crystal clear and irrefutable—the foods that cross our lips have a profound and lasting impact on all aspects of our health. Thankfully, it's as simple as the choice between right and wrong. The right foods like fruits, vegetables, whole grains, oily fish and nuts prevent disease and give us life, while the wrong foods like sugary beverages, fast foods, and junk foods promote disease and reduce vitality. I know what ends up in your cupboards and your fridge is dictated by what you put in your grocery cart, so I am on a mission to provide you with the grocery shopping education you need to ensure that your cart gets filled with the right foods for a healthy life.

In the pages that follow, I am going to arm you with a road map for healthy grocery shopping that will place you and your loved ones on the fast track to nutritional excellence. I am determined to help you fully experience the awesome benefits that healthy, home-prepared foods can provide and understand that the first step is putting the right foods in the grocery cart. I am also fully aware of how overwhelming and frankly daunting healthy grocery shopping can seem. With up to 40,000 food choices including 100 different cereals and 50 different yogurts available to choose from, it's a wonder that even the most motivated and knowledgeable healthy shoppers can triumph. But have no fear! I am here to ensure your success. As a nutrition expert, wife, and mother of four that has been grocery shopping for three decades, I have gotten it down to a science that you too can apply and succeed with.

My guidance and instructions promise to be straightforward, clear, prescriptive and in some cases profoundly liberating. Over the years in my private wellness coaching practice, I have taken my pupils through the grocery store to instruct them in healthy food selections. I call these sessions my "grocery clinics," and they have been proven to dramatically improve the nutritional health of those I mentor. Consider this chapter your grocery clinic. Your first step should be to commit the "golden rules" for healthy eating to memory before your next trip to the supermarket. They are the bedrock for nutritional success and can easily be mastered in a short period of time. For optimal success, take the information that follows with you to the grocery store until you have mastered the task. Follow the "ground rules" provided for each basic area of the grocery store until you feel like you have it down pat, and of course, use my list of Dr. Ann approved foods to keep things fail safe. I want you to take complete advantage of the detailed shopping lists I have conveniently provided to be sure you are stocking up on the right foods and avoiding the wrong ones. Eventually, you will not need my written guidance because knowledge of the fundamental "ground rules" will become second nature, and you will automatically apply them as the basis for all the foods that go into your shopping cart. Lastly, because I want nothing less than the very best nourishment for you and your family, I promise that if you follow my guidance that is exactly what you will get.

The Golden Rules Of
HEALTHY EATING

Enjoy:

- ➤ A wealth of fruits and veggies, especially the "superstars"
- ➤ Monounsaturated fats as your main fats—extra virgin olive oil, canola oil, nuts, seeds, and avocados
- ➤ 100% whole grains—at least three servings a day
- ➤ Omega 3 fats regularly— oily fish, omega 3 eggs, canola oil, walnuts, flax seeds, dark leafy greens, and whole soy foods
- ➤ Any variety of beans—on a daily basis is best
- ➤ Healthy protein at each meal—fish, shellfish, poultry, low fat or skim dairy products, nuts, seeds, beans, whole soy foods, and omega 3 eggs
- ➤ Make water your primary beverage

Restrict/Avoid:

- ➤ "Great White Hazards"— white flour products like white bread, white rice, white potatoes, and sugar/sweets
- ➤ Saturated fats—fatty cuts of red meat, whole dairy products, butter, and palm oil
- ➤ Trans fats—strictly avoid this group, which includes stick margarine, processed foods containing partially hydrogenated oils, and shortening
- ➤ Red meat, especially processed and fatty varieties—Limit red meat to two servings or less weekly
- ➤ Sugary beverages—soda, fruit drinks, sports drinks, vitamin waters, etc.

> *"A massive amount of meticulous consumer behavior research has gone into creating the grocery store layout that results in the most sales and the highest profits."*

Reality Check

Grocery stores are in the business of selling foods for maximum profits—not improving your health. This is a critically important concept to grasp because, with few exceptions, the foods that have the biggest profit margins are the unhealthiest like sodas, pastries, and chips. It is precisely these two opposing forces—what is best for grocery stores versus what is best for human health—that creates the confusion and bewilderment consumers feel when trying to decipher which foods are good for them and which foods are bad. In the pages that follow, I promise to clear away this dense fog of confusion so you can readily and easily make the right choices.

Before we begin, I want you to get a sense of how the grocery stores' quest for profits can create powerful challenges for "healthy" grocery shopping, especially in those who are uninformed or naïve to this reality. Relentless and potent marketing forces are at play throughout the grocery store to lure you to buy food, especially those that bring the biggest profits. Have you ever noticed how consistent the layout of one grocery store is to another? Indeed, even among competing chains, the aisles display an uncanny degree of uniformity. This is not mere happenstance. A massive amount of meticulous consumer behavior research has gone into creating the grocery store layout that results in the most sales and the highest profits. To illustrate, let me share a few common strategies. Staple items like eggs and milk that comprise the most frequent grocery store purchases are almost always placed towards the back of the grocery store. This placement forces you to walk past hundreds of other food products that grocers hope you will decide to buy along the way. Sections nearest the entrance to the store are the preferred locations for "sensory

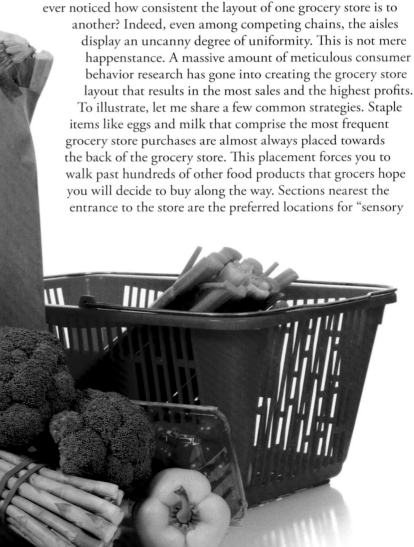

rich" items. These are the products that exploit our automatic attraction to powerful sensory stimuli like the vivid colors of fresh flowers, the aroma of freshly brewed coffee (notice the coffee shops popping up just inside your grocer's front door) or the irresistible scent of freshly baked goods. Grocers know that the more intense the sensory stimuli the more likely we will buy on impulse. Impulse buys are the proverbial "icing on the cake" for supermarkets. And how about those obtrusive, practically knock-you-over displays placed in high profile areas like the end of aisles or just as you walk in through the grocer's front doors? These spots are prime real estate and are logically reserved for foods with the highest profit margins (nutritionally anemic, processed junk foods) and the ones we notoriously tend to grab on a whim. I can recall walking into a supermarket a few years back to be met at the entrance by an almost majestic display of junk foods. There was literally a floor to ceiling archway of bags of potato chips and cases of soda that you had to enter followed by an almost enclosed circular arrangement of assorted boxes of cookies and donuts. It was like entering a junk food carnival. I could go on, but what I want you to really grasp is that where and how grocery stores display products is a highly researched, proven science used to encourage you to buy as much food as possible and make them the greatest profits. Let me warn you again that for the most part, the most lucrative sales are for the wrong foods—the ones that promote chronic diseases like diabetes, obesity, and heart disease. Don't give in to these ploys!

You Have The Power!

It is my hope, now that you are armed with the awareness that a supermarket's main interest is in making money and not your health, you will feel compelled to always shop with a strong sense of personal empowerment and a deeply committed purpose. Only YOU should be in control of the foods that go into your cart, not the manipulative forces of grocery store marketing. Make a concerted effort to tell yourself each and every time you walk through the supermarket front doors that you will remain strong and steadfast in selecting foods that are good for you and your family (which I will carefully outline for you in the upcoming sections). Stand tall and remain proactive with every step down every aisle and do not succumb to the marketing forces that push you to make unhealthy (not on Dr. Ann's list!) choices. Learn to consciously shut it all out like I do. No giving in to your senses! No impulse buying! No extraneous purchases! No wrong foods in your cart! Make a mental, or better yet, a written pact with you and your loved ones that everything that goes into your grocery cart will emanate from you and only you. You are the nutritional gatekeeper of your family, and your selections should always be in the best interests of their health and well-being.

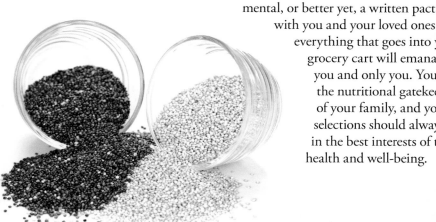

Attitude Adjustment

Before we get into the grocery store, I have some final wisdom that I know will make the process more pleasant and more successful. Everything is easier when we are happy, so I urge you to develop a positive mental attitude! I cannot stress enough how important it is to nurture and cultivate a joyful, cheery frame of mind relative to your grocery shopping duties. The reason for this all-important attitude adjustment is elemental—it simply makes no sense to loathe an activity that is required for health. Make no mistake—you and your family's chances of achieving and maintaining good health without regularly eating home-prepared meals is near impossible. Within our modern food culture, you simply cannot rely on the foods or meals someone else has provided—from convenience stores or restaurants—and expect good health. In fact—expect the opposite. Studies consistently show that home-prepared meals provide more of the good, health-promoting stuff like fruits, vegetables, fiber and essential nutrients while restaurant-based meals provide more (and in many cases way more) of the disease-promoting stuff like excess calories, sodium, refined carbs, unhealthy fats and sugar. Thankfully, there are a host of sound reasons why you should be positive and upbeat about your grocery shopping opportunities.

➤ It can definitely be gentler on your wallet. A significant portion of your food dollars spent in a restaurant or fast food joint go toward non-food related expenses like labor and manufacturing.

➤ As noted above, grocery shopping offers a profound opportunity to improve your family's health, especially if you are the "nutritional gatekeeper" for your household. According to the experts, about 72 percent of what crosses the lips of family members is under the direct control of a single individual. This is the individual who does most of the grocery shopping and meal preparations, and in about 90 percent of households it is the same individual, AKA the nutritional gatekeeper. For me, the nutritional gatekeeper of my household, I consider grocery shopping a labor of love. I urge you to cultivate this same belief and promise it will warm your heart.

➤ Healthy food choices abound. Never before has there been such a dazzling array of healthy choices in the standard grocer. Whether it is tapping into the goodness of whole grains or the stunning variety of brightly colored fruits and veggies—disease-busting, life-saving selections are more bountiful than ever.

➤ It provides an opportunity to get some "lifestyle exercise." Grocery shopping includes a bit of walking, pushing, pulling, and lifting. Fortunately, this movement can make a meaningful contribution to your body's innate requirement for regular physical activity. In my grocery store, I am well known by the baggers as the lady who makes you thread her arms with as many shopping bags as possible to avoid using the cart and never wants help to her car. I do this because I know it is a very efficient way for me to simultaneously get some resistance and aerobic exercise during my shopping trips.

➤ It offers some cognitive exercise too. Using your intellectual capacities to compare prices, calculate savings, or decipher food labels is good for your brain.

➤ Grocery shopping offers a social outlet. We are inherently social beings and require interaction with others for good health, especially mental health. The grocery store can be a common place to run into friends and neighbors. Whether you simply extend a warm smile or engage in a full conversation, the social connection is good for you.

> ❝Grocery shopping includes a bit of walking, pushing, pulling, and lifting. Fortunately, this movement can make a meaningful contribution to your body's innate requirement for regular physical activity.❞

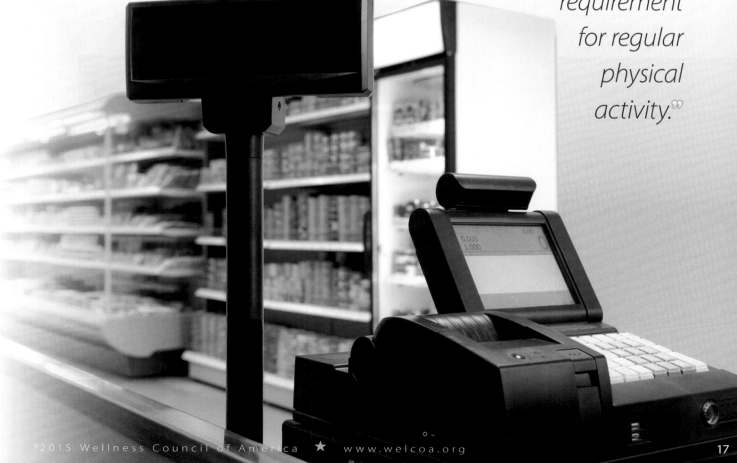

Dr. Ann's...
WHAT'S FOR DINNER?

One day, years back when I was juggling a busy medical practice with raising four young children and putting a tasty, healthy, husband-happy meal on the table each night, I had a revelation. I recognized that the hard part of cooking dinner was figuring out what I was going to make and having the proper ingredients readily available in my kitchen.

And the light bulb went off. I realized that if I had ten or so dinner meal plans that I knew satisfied my criteria for health and taste, along with the ingredients that comprised them, grocery shopping and preparing dinner would be so much easier and less taxing. And so I did it.

I spent a Saturday morning writing down fifteen dinner meal plans and their ingredients on one side of fifteen separate 3 × 5 index cards. If I did not know the recipe by rote memory, I wrote it down on the flip side of the index card. I laminated the index cards at the Kinko's down the street, punched a hole in the top left corner of each, and put them all onto a simple O ring. This handy, makeshift "Dinner Menus and Recipe Booklet" became my constant pocketbook companion and my secret weapon for de-stressing family dinner.

In fact, I found my portable, compact dinner guide so helpful—I created one suitable for the marketplace. I call it *What's for Dinner... 15 Healthy, Family-Friendly Meal Plans and Recipes.* You can own this convenient tool too, which is available at:

www.DrAnnWellness.com

Before You Go

In addition to putting on that happy face and feeling good about your upcoming grocery shopping experience, here are a few additional before-you-go tips that will help you.

1. Do not shop hungry. The hungrier you are, the more likely you will be tempted to place high-risk, unhealthy foods like sweets and junk foods into your shopping cart. Because of what transpires in our brains in a state of hunger, we simply lose self-control, especially when surrounded by a large variety of tempting foods that are just an arm's length away. Take the edge off your hunger by eating a "smart" pre-shopping snack as needed. For best results, choose something with a little healthy fat, some protein, and some fiber. My top picks would be a small handful of nuts, some baby carrots dipped in hummus, or a few apple slices spread with a bit of peanut butter.

2. Beware of the pitfalls of shopping with young children. For those of you, like me, who have had to grocery shop with young children in tow, you already know that it slows things down (which is great for the grocery stores) and frequently creates a more stressful shopping experience. What you may not recognize is that those little ones can become a powerful force in terms of unhealthy foods piling up in the grocery cart. The reason is fundamental and human—"the whine factor" works! And boy do the grocery stores know it. Resisting the pleas, cries and at times, full on temper tantrums flowing from a child's mouth when they "want that food" is extremely challenging. It is human nature to give in. You may have noticed that the kid-friendly junk foods— think pre-packed "lunches," sugary cereals, and candy are on the lower tiers of the grocery shelves. Grocers are well aware that if the little ones can see it they will want it and beg you for it if they have to. Over the past decade, grocery stores have become increasingly kid-friendly with the likes of free cookies (ugh, even in the age of the childhood obesity epidemic!) and kiddie-sized shopping carts because it is good business for them. Beware however, these gimmicks may not be what are best for you or your small children.

3. Shop with a list. I cannot overstate the power of this practice. Carving out a little time to sit down and plan out your family meals so you can create a shopping list has numerous benefits. First and foremost, it provides a safeguard against impulse purchases that can boost what you pay at checkout and sabotage your good health. Impulse purchases are notorious for high-risk foods. Shopping lists help to ensure that your kitchen will be stocked with the foods and ingredients your family needs for upcoming meals, and save you wasteful trips back to the grocery store.

Preparing a shopping list can also streamline the shopping experience, and help you get in and out more quickly (remember the more time you spend in the grocery store the more likely you will pick up foods that you don't need). Last, but not least, it forces you to plan your meals ahead of time, which dramatically increases the likelihood that you will actually prepare them. To make healthy meal planning a snap, be sure to check out my *Eat Right for Life®: Cookbook Companion.*

4. If you use them (and I hope you do), don't forget to bring your reusable, eco-friendly shopping bags. This will help reduce your own family's carbon footprint and reduce pollution. Plastic shopping bags require oil to produce and are non-biodegradable. Although they are recyclable, unfortunately most end up in our oceans and landfills as refuse. Aside from being green, eco-friendly shopping bags accommodate more food, are more comfortable and easier to carry, and can ultimately bring down the cost of your groceries. Some stores even provide a small credit for shoppers that provide their own bags. Otherwise, the less plastic bags you use at checkout, the lower the grocer's overhead and the more savings they can pass on to you.

5. Think ahead for safe transport of your groceries from the store to your kitchen. In some cases, you may need to have a cooler in your car. According to food safety experts, any perishable food should be refrigerated within two hours. If the outside temperature exceeds 90 degrees F, you will need to get perishable foods home and in the freezer or fridge more quickly—within one hour. If your supermarket is more than 30 minutes away from your home or if you know that your trip home from the grocery store will be delayed by more than 30 minutes for errands or such, pack a cooler. Place any meat, seafood, poultry or eggs in it to safeguard against the growth of harmful bacteria that could cause a food borne illness.

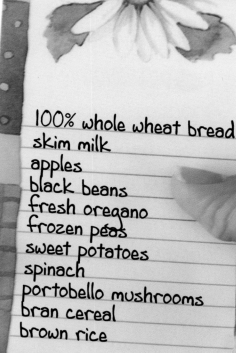

100% whole wheat bread
skim milk
apples
black beans
fresh oregano
frozen peas
sweet potatoes
spinach
portobello mushrooms
bran cereal
brown rice

Dr. Ann Recommends...
MAKING THE LIST!

Always keep your grocery list in a prominent, visible place on your kitchen counter with a pen or pencil handy. Encourage your family members to jot down things they may need and be sure to write down those must-have kitchen staples before they run out.

"*Focus on selecting whole, real, unprocessed foods. These are the foods generously provided by Mother Nature—'foods as found and foods as grown.' These humble, yet all-mighty foods do not come in glitzy boxes or packages complete with an ingredients list boasting strange, chemical-like words.*"

General Guidance

We are just about to begin our virtual grocery tour, which is the perfect time to make note of some very important general guidance that can dramatically simplify our journey.

1. Focus on selecting whole, real, unprocessed foods. These are the foods generously provided by Mother Nature—"foods as found and foods as grown." These humble, yet all-mighty foods do not come in glitzy boxes or packages complete with an ingredients list boasting strange, chemical-like words. Rather, they are as simple and tasty as their names suggest, and come in a delicious array of options, including apples, pears, kale, cabbage, brown rice, oatmeal, fish and chicken. As an easy and reliable "filter" for making real food selections, ask yourself if the food is something that your great, great grandfather could have eaten before you put it in your cart. Although there are notable exceptions, much of the time if the answer is "no", the selection will not be good for you.

2. Concentrate your shopping around the periphery of the store. In most all grocery outlets, the whole, real foods will be found in the perimeter aisles. Conversely, the interior aisles are home to the seemingly endless displays of factory-made, processed foods that I want you to minimize or avoid.

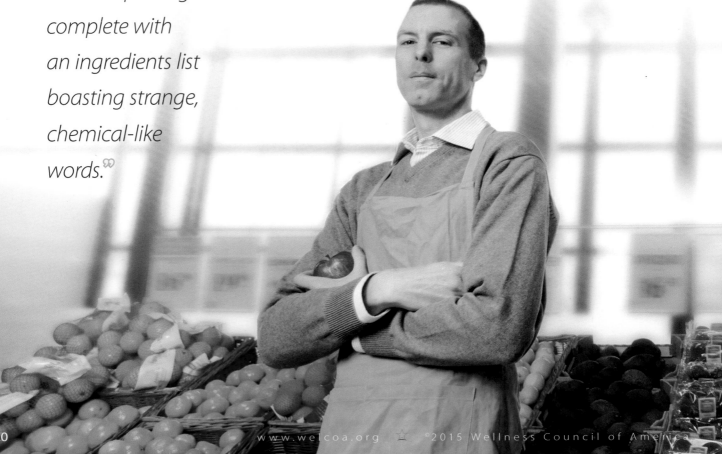

3. Beware of dubious health claims. Do not get sucked in by the in-your-face healthy phrases like "contains whole grains" or "trans-fat free" that boldly shout out from the front of packages. With very rare exceptions, these claims are a reliable indicator of a man-made, not nature-made, food. Even worse, many of these foods are the ones that are bad for you. Classic examples include packaged chips and donuts that promote "trans-fat free" or toaster pastries boasting, "contains whole grains." Do not be duped by these slick packaging ploys. Having taken lots of nutritionally naïve consumers through the grocery aisles—this is one of the most common mistakes I see them make.

4. If you do reach for a packaged product, quickly vet its ingredients list before putting it in your shopping buggy. While abiding by the suggestions above pretty much takes care of this one, just say no to it if:

   ➤ **It contains words you have a hard time pronouncing or that are foreign to you.** Steer clear of foods that list ingredients that read as if they were something from Frankenstein's lab like "butylated hydroxyanisole" or "acelsulfame-K."

   ➤ **The ingredients list is long.** My general rule of thumb is to stick to those with lists of less than seven ingredients. Although there will be some exceptions, like cereals and "healthy" packaged foods like hummus or salsa, the overwhelming majority of the foods on my master, "Dr. Ann Approved Foods" shopping list have less than seven ingredients. Most will have less than four.

   ➤ **It has any of the following words: partially hydrogenated, fully hydrogenated, shortening, artificial color(s), artificial flavor(s), or high fructose corn syrup (HFCS).** While some may signify the presence of truly toxic compounds like trans fats (partially hydrogenated oils), they are all telling markers for contrived products of modern food technology versus real food.

Dr. Ann's Tip...
JOIN A CSA!

CSA stands for "community supported agriculture" and thankfully, this new system for procuring farm fresh local produce is becoming more and more accessible. As a member of a CSA, you pay an upfront subscription to a local farm to receive a weekly or biweekly box of fresh produce. Before I had my own vegetable garden, I used a CSA and loved it. I highly recommend them, and hope they'll inspire you to start your own garden, too!

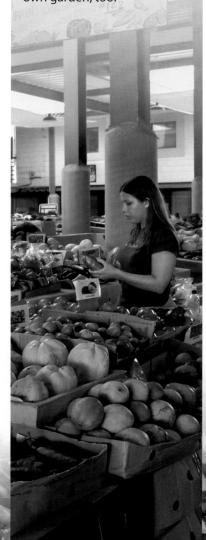

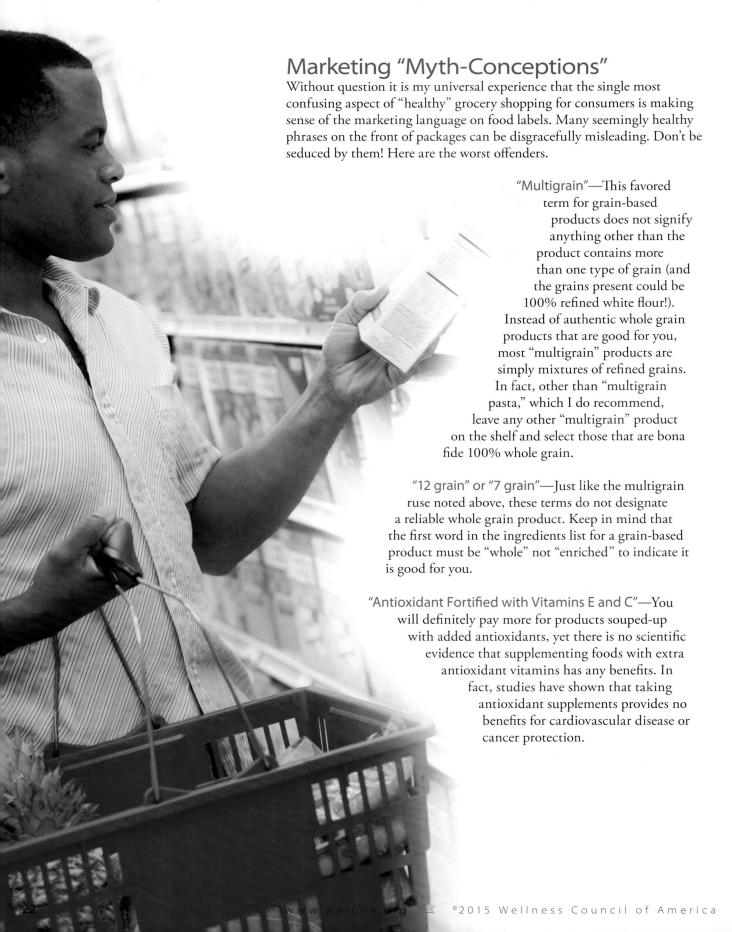

Marketing "Myth-Conceptions"

Without question it is my universal experience that the single most confusing aspect of "healthy" grocery shopping for consumers is making sense of the marketing language on food labels. Many seemingly healthy phrases on the front of packages can be disgracefully misleading. Don't be seduced by them! Here are the worst offenders.

"Multigrain"—This favored term for grain-based products does not signify anything other than the product contains more than one type of grain (and the grains present could be 100% refined white flour!). Instead of authentic whole grain products that are good for you, most "multigrain" products are simply mixtures of refined grains. In fact, other than "multigrain pasta," which I do recommend, leave any other "multigrain" product on the shelf and select those that are bona fide 100% whole grain.

"12 grain" or "7 grain"—Just like the multigrain ruse noted above, these terms do not designate a reliable whole grain product. Keep in mind that the first word in the ingredients list for a grain-based product must be "whole" not "enriched" to indicate it is good for you.

"Antioxidant Fortified with Vitamins E and C"—You will definitely pay more for products souped-up with added antioxidants, yet there is no scientific evidence that supplementing foods with extra antioxidant vitamins has any benefits. In fact, studies have shown that taking antioxidant supplements provides no benefits for cardiovascular disease or cancer protection.

"Organic" on processed food packages—Unfortunately, studies repeatedly show that consumers believe foods with "organic" on their labels are more nutritious and less likely to cause weight gain. This is simply not true. "Organic" simply signifies that the food was produced without pesticides, antibiotics or growth hormones. There are oodles of processed "organic" foods on grocery shelves that are loaded with calories, refined flour, salt, unhealthy fats and excess sugar— so be careful!

"Made with real fruit"—This is a common phrase for packages of toaster pastries and pancakes, and it simply means that "some" fruit (typically fruit juice) is present. Unfortunately, "some" is usually a tiny, nutritionally-irrelevant amount. On at least one brand of toaster pastries, salt is listed before the fruit on the ingredients list. In other words, the product contains more salt by weight than real fruit—not good!

"High in fiber"—Because of the sparkling and well-deserved healthy reputation of dietary fiber, this three-word phrase is literally all over the place now. It means that a single serving of the food provides at least five grams of fiber, but that does not necessarily translate to any health benefits. With few exceptions, products that list "high in fiber" are manufactured foods in which isolated fiber— commonly maltodextrin, inulin (also called chicory root), oat fiber, and wheat fiber—have been artificially added to it. At this point in science, there is no evidence for any health benefits from eating isolated forms of fiber. This is in stark contrast to the fiber that is naturally a part of whole grains, beans, fruits and vegetables. So forget the processed and go for the real!

"A full serving of vegetables"—For me, this one is a personal pet peeve and a blatant give-away that the food is factory-made. Get your vegetables from the real thing and forget the fruit drinks, crackers, chips, and sauces that unfairly take advantage of vegetables' virtues to entice you to buy their products.

"All natural"—This is one of the most common claims on processed food products and it is essentially meaningless. You find it plastered all over "unnatural" products like sugary beverages and chips. Even meats that have been artificially injected with salt solutions can bear this misleading designation. Completely ignore this deceptive term.

Nutrition Fac

Serving Size   1 Cup (53g/
Servings Per Container   A

Amount Per Serving

Calories 190   Calories fror

                                    % Dail

Total Fat 3g

   Saturated Fat 0g

   Trans Fat 0g

Cholesterol 0mg

Sodium 100mg

Potassium 300mg

Total Carbohydrate 37g

   Dietary Fiber 8g

      Soluble Fiber

      Insoluble Fibe

   Sugars 13g

Protein 9g

Vitamin A 0%

      4%

Now, Let's Go Shopping!

FRESH PRODUCE

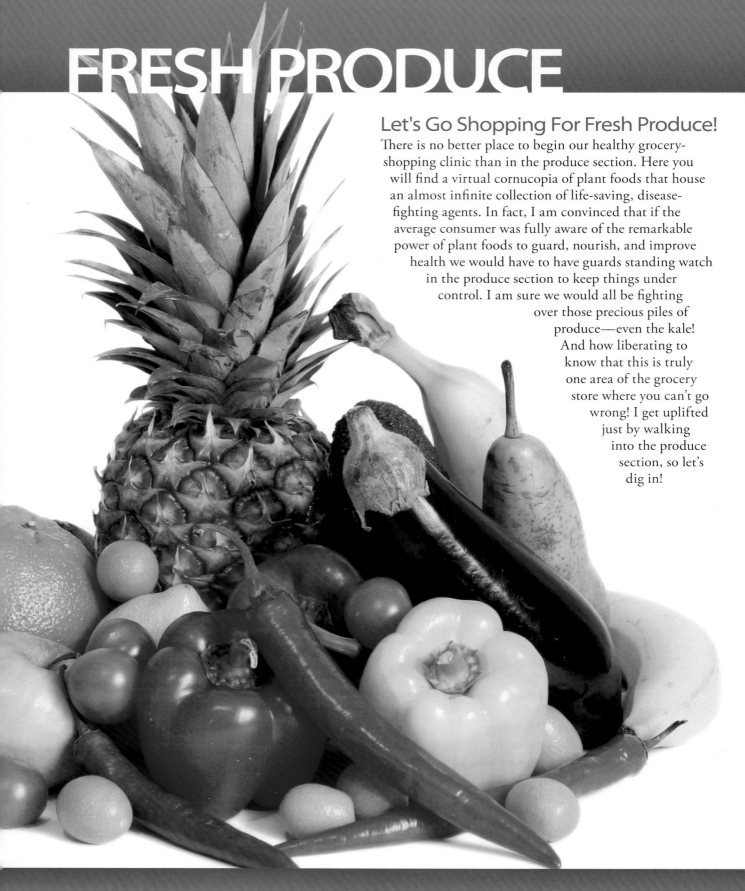

Let's Go Shopping For Fresh Produce!

There is no better place to begin our healthy grocery-shopping clinic than in the produce section. Here you will find a virtual cornucopia of plant foods that house an almost infinite collection of life-saving, disease-fighting agents. In fact, I am convinced that if the average consumer was fully aware of the remarkable power of plant foods to guard, nourish, and improve health we would have to have guards standing watch in the produce section to keep things under control. I am sure we would all be fighting over those precious piles of produce—even the kale! And how liberating to know that this is truly one area of the grocery store where you can't go wrong! I get uplifted just by walking into the produce section, so let's dig in!

Ground Rules

➤ **Variety.** The greater the variety of produce you eat, the healthier you will be.

➤ **Deep rich color.** The pigments in plant foods that impart their stunning colors also have stunning health-boosting power. From the bright red of the tomato's lycopene to the deep purple of berries' anthocyanins—take full advantage of theses sensational agents by choosing lots of deeply colored produce.

➤ **Quantity.** This is simple math—your refrigerator and fruit bowl will need to be brimming with produce for you and your family to succeed in getting the recommended seven to nine daily servings. Trust me—you will never know just how healthy and alive you can feel until you have done this.

➤ **Concentrate on the superstars.** Although all forms of fresh produce have beneficial nutrients to offer, some are simply stellar. These are noted as "superstars."

➤ **Think convenience as needed.** If saving time in the kitchen is especially important to you, make note of the growing selections of convenient, ready-to-eat items like bagged salad greens, shredded cabbage, chopped bell peppers, "baby" carrots, and sliced apples. (But be aware that you will generally pay more for these labor saving selections).

➤ **Look for "locally grown" produce.** Locally sourced fruits and veggies will typically be cheaper, fresher, and tastier, and it is definitely better for your local economy and the environment.

➤ **Unless you are lean and active, restrict white potatoes.** As a population, we consume a disproportionate share of our "veggies" from this starch. The flesh of a white potato is very rapidly digested, giving rise to sudden and high elevations of blood glucose that can have adverse metabolic effects. In this regard, the best choice would be small new potatoes and the worst would be large russet potatoes.

➤ **Smaller is healthier.** Because the nutritional goodness of produce concentrates in and just under its skin, you would be wise to go for the smallest varieties offered for produce where the skin is commonly consumed. The smaller the piece of produce (think apples, berries, tomatoes), the higher its skin to flesh ratio, and the better it will be for you.

"12" AND "15"

Although the benefits of conventionally grown fruits and veggies far outweigh health risks for pesticides, you may find it useful to know which forms of produce are the dirtiest (have the highest concentration of pesticides) and which are the cleanest.

According to the Environmental Working Group (EWG), a national not-for-profit devoted to informing consumers about pesticide exposure and risks, here are the "dirty dozen" and "cleanest fifteen."

Dirty Dozen:
1. Apples
2. Celery
3. Strawberries
4. Peaches
5. Spinach
6. Nectarines—imported
7. Grapes—imported
8. Sweet bell peppers
9. Potatoes
10. Blueberries—domestic
11. Lettuce
12. Kale/collard greens

Cleanest Fifteen:
1. Onions
2. Sweet corn
3. Pineapples
4. Avocado
5. Asparagus
6. Sweet peas
7. Mangoes
8. Eggplant
9. Cantaloupe—domestic
10. Kiwi
11. Cabbage
12. Watermelon
13. Sweet potatoes
14. Grapefruit
15. Mushrooms

FRESH PRODUCE

Shopping List
(Everything on this list is a superstar food!)

✓ Any form of dark leafy greens: dark lettuce greens (arugula, spinach, mesclun, water cress, romaine, bibb, etc.), kale, collard greens, mustard greens, turnip greens, Swiss chard

✓ Any member of the cruciferous family of veggies: broccoli, cabbage (all varieties), cauliflower, Brussels sprouts, broccoli rabe

✓ The allium family: onions, scallions, shallots, leeks, garlic

✓ Bell peppers: red, orange, yellow and green

✓ Deep orange veggies: carrots, sweet potatoes, winter squash

✓ Other veggie superstars: tomatoes, asparagus, sprouts (especially brocco sprouts), avocados

✓ Mushrooms: all varieties

✓ Fresh herbs: all varieties; fresh ginger root

✓ Berries: all varieties

✓ Apples: all varieties

✓ Any whole citrus: oranges, grapefruit, tangerines, lemons, limes, etc.

✓ Melon: cantaloupe, watermelon

✓ Other superstar fruits: kiwi, mango, papaya, pineapple, apricots, pears, pomegranate, peaches, plums, cherries, red/purple grapes, guava

✓ Fresh prepared salsa and guacamole (both are super-healthy and are usually located in the produce section)

Dr. Ann's Tip!
Strive to have a serving from each of the following daily: dark leafy greens (raw or cooked), cruciferous veggies, whole citrus and berries.

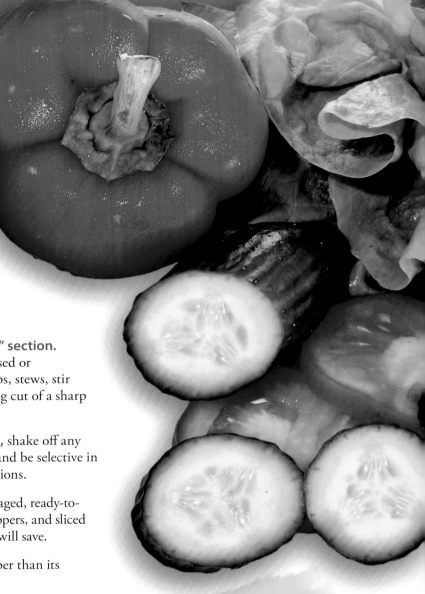

Produce Best Bargains

➤ **Look for "locally grown" or "in season" signs.** They are usually a better bargain, fresher and tastier.

➤ **Buy in bulk.** Purchasing large bags of apples, oranges, onions, etc. can save you up to 40% versus purchasing them individually, but be sure to eat them before they go bad.

➤ **Go for the store specials.** If you can, check out the in-store specials in your paper or online before you go and plan your needs (and grocery list) accordingly.

➤ **Be sure to check out the "reduced produce" section.** Here you will find dramatic reductions on bruised or blemished produce that can be just fine for soups, stews, stir frys, and smoothies—or with the discriminating cut of a sharp paring knife.

➤ **For produce that is priced based on weight,** shake off any residual water left from the on-shelf sprinklers and be selective in choosing the produce with the most edible portions.

➤ **Be aware that you will pay more** for pre-packaged, ready-to-eat items like lettuce, baby carrots, diced bell peppers, and sliced apples. If you clean, slice, and dice yourself, you will save.

➤ **Keep in mind** that fresh produce is often cheaper than its frozen counter part.

Dr. Ann Recommends...
FOR WEIGHT LOSS

If you are watching your weight or trying to lose weight, avoid:

➤ Dried fruit with the exception of apricots

➤ Tropical fruits—bananas, pineapple, mango and papaya

➤ White potatoes

These foods will kick up your blood sugar level more so than other produce choices, which can hamper your efforts to lose weight.

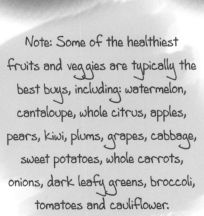

Note: Some of the healthiest fruits and veggies are typically the best buys, including: watermelon, cantaloupe, whole citrus, apples, pears, kiwi, plums, grapes, cabbage, sweet potatoes, whole carrots, onions, dark leafy greens, broccoli, tomatoes and cauliflower.

MEATS & SEAFOOD

Let's Go Shopping For Meats And Seafood!

Including some "healthy" protein at mealtime is an essential component of optimal nutrition. Learning how to find your way in the meat and seafood section of the grocery store can make the difference between good health and bad health, so adhere to the following directions in order to take advantage of the good and leave the bad behind.

Ground Rules

➤ **Restrict red meats (beef, pork, lamb), especially fatty cuts and processed varieties.**

- Limit read meat to two servings or less weekly.
- Avoid processed meats—bacon, sausage, ham, hot dogs, salami, etc. Avoid fatty cuts—ribs, rib eyes, briskets, porter house, T-bones, and standard ground meat.

➤ **Choose ground turkey breast or ground chicken breast as a healthier choice than standard ground beef.**

➤ **If ground beef is a must, choose ground sirloin, ground round, or extra lean ground beef.**

➤ **When you choose red meat, select the leanest cuts.** The leanest varieties are the one with less white portions ("marbling" created by saturated fats) and more red portions (muscle protein). Look for cuts containing the words loin or round to make wise selections. The terms lean and extra lean can also help you choose less fatty options.

➤ **Choose lean poultry as a healthier alternative to red meat.**

➤ **Focus on seafood.** The superstars in this section provide high quality protein along with healthy omega 3 fats.

Know Your Grades.

The grade of meat signifies its fat content. "Select" is the leanest grade (7% fat), followed by choice (15% to 35% fat), and then prime (35% to 45% fat).

Dr. Ann's Tips...
FOR SELECTING MEAT

Be Careful in Selecting Your Ground Poultry

Ground poultry like "ground turkey" can have just as much fat as standard ground beef. Always choose ground turkey breast or ground chicken breast. They provide the least fat and calories. Many brands are 99% fat-free.

Shopping List

✓ Fish, especially the oily varieties that provide an abundance of omega 3 fats—salmon, herring, trout, tuna, halibut. Wild Alaskan Salmon is my top pick. Avoid shark, marlin, tilefish, king mackerel, and swordfish due to toxins. Young children and women of childbearing years should avoid fresh tuna due to methyl mercury.

✓ Any shellfish—clams, shrimp, oysters, lobster, mussels, scallops, crawfish and crab.

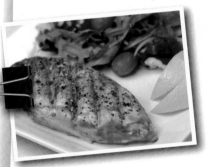

✓ Poultry—any cut of turkey or chicken. Skinless options and white (breast) meat have the least fat. Ground turkey breast or ground chicken breast are also great options.

✓ Chicken sausage—several brands are available that are low in fat and free of potentially dangerous nitrates, like Casual Gourmet, Aiddell's and Al Fresco.

✓ Lean beef—Eye round, top round, round tip, top sirloin, flank steak, and bottom round cuts. Extra lean (93%-96%) ground beef. Veal cutlets. If grass fed beef is available and affordable for you, it is a healthier and tastier alternative.

✓ Lean pork—Tenderloin is the best choice followed by boneless loin roast and boneless loin chops.

SALMON
Farm Raised vs. Wild Salmon

One of the most frequently asked questions I receive when engaging with a live audience is, "What about farmed raised salmon versus wild salmon?"

About 70 percent of the fresh salmon consumed in America comes from farm raised salmon (also known as Atlantic salmon). Although farm raised salmon is chock full of heart-healthy omega 3 fats that can make a very positive contribution to overall health, its wild counterpart is superior. Both have comparable amounts of omega 3 fats, but farm raised salmon has more unhealthy saturated fats, a much higher omega 6: omega 3 ratio (which is not good), and can contain traces of antibiotics and environmental contaminants like PCBs and dioxins.

Fresh wild salmon is typically only available from early summer to late fall, but you can usually find it frozen, and you can always find it canned. Wild salmon is always my first choice for health and taste.

Make note that farmed salmon from South America (usually Chile) and Washington State is usually the "cleanest," while that from northern Europe (Scotland) is usually the dirtiest. Removing the skin before eating is another strategy for reducing your exposure to PCBs and dioxins.

DAIRY & EGGS

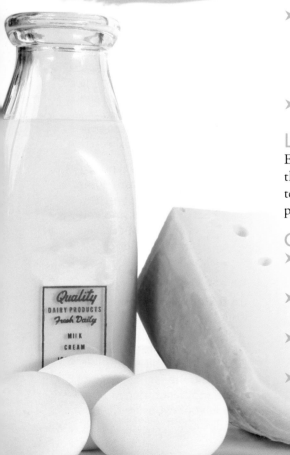

Sweet Tips For Healthy Yogurt

Since the only yogurt I recommend is plain, here is my best advice for healthfully sweetening your plain yogurt.

✓ Blend it with some berries or fresh cut up fruit of your choice.

✓ Add 1-2 teaspoons of honey, maple syrup, or molasses.

✓ Mix equal portions of vanilla and plain yogurt (½ vanilla and ½ plain).

✓ Add 1-2 teaspoons of a berry-based fruit spread.

Let's Go Shopping For Dairy!

Just like the meat/seafood section, the dairy case is a mixed bag. Some selections will enhance your health, while others can definitely work against you. With the directions that follow, your future trips in the dairy section should go from mass confusion to simple, easy, and totally liberating success, especially when it comes to grabbing the right yogurt.

Ground Rules

➤ Avoid full-fat dairy products.

➤ Avoid whole milk (exception: children two and younger), full-fat cheeses, ice creams, cream, sour cream, and butter. They are loaded with artery-clogging saturated fat and excess calories.

➤ Always choose low-fat, reduced-fat, or skim versions of dairy products.

➤ For dairy products that you consume regularly, especially daily like yogurt or milk—choose organic varieties.

➤ Select the one and only truly healthy yogurt—low-fat or non-fat plain. Most flavored yogurts, especially the kid-friendly brands (Go-Gurt, Danimals) are filled with added sugars. In most cases, more than a standard dessert. In fact, you should consider flavored yogurt a dessert.

➤ Avoid all stick margarines.

Let's Go Shopping For Eggs!

Eggs are an underappreciated source of high-quality, inexpensive protein that comes along with several other key nutrients. Thanks to modern food technology, some eggs are healthier than ever because they provide those precious omega 3 fats, DHA and EPA.

Ground Rules

➤ Select those fortified with omega 3 fats. Look for "omega 3" or "DHA" on the label.

➤ Recognize that "free-range" does not always indicate the presence of omega 3 fats.

➤ Know that there is no nutritional difference between white eggs and brown eggs.

➤ If you are diabetic, have high cholesterol, or have cardiovascular disease, enjoy up to four eggs a week. Healthy folks need not limit eggs.

SHOPPING LIST

✓ Plain cows milk—skim or 1%. Organic is best. Avoid flavored milks.

✓ Organic plain soy milk. Avoid flavored versions.

✓ Lactose-free skim or 1% milk—for those lactose intolerant.

✓ Low-fat or non-fat plain yogurt. I prefer Greek style like Oikos for its creamy texture and robust protein levels. Organic is best. Large cartons are best buy.

✓ Low-fat or non-fat vanilla yogurt (for those who want to mix with plain for added sweetness). Avoid all the other flavored yogurts, especially those marketed to children. Avoid artificially sweetened yogurts.

✓ Park skim or reduced fat (made with 2% milk) cheeses—part skim mozzarella, 2% milk cheddar, Swiss, or provolone.

✓ Low-fat or fat-free cottage cheese/ricotta cheese.

✓ Fat-free, light or low-fat sour cream.

✓ Fat-free or reduced fat cream cheese.

✓ Light spreadable cheeses—Boursin Light, Alouette Light or Rondele Light brands are good choices.

✓ Highly flavored cheeses—feta, parmesan, and goat (in moderation).

✓ Trans fat-free margarine spreads—Smart Balance, Promise, Country Crock, Olivio brands. Light varieties have fewer calories.

✓ Whole soy foods—tofu and tempeh (frequently found in the dairy section).

✓ Omega-3 fortified eggs—Eggland's Best, Nature's Design, Egg Sense, and Born Free are available brands.

DAIRY

I Choose Organic Dairy Products

Dairy products are derived from cows, which exist at the tip top of the food chain, so you must consider excessive exposure to potentially harmful environmental contaminants like heavy metals, PCBs, dioxins, antibiotics and pesticides. As edible species move up the food chain, harmful environmental chemicals can naturally bio-concentrate. Additionally, many of these compounds are fat-soluble and tend to build up in the fats that are a natural part of dairy foods. (Which is another reason to choose lower fat dairy!) Frequent, recurrent exposures to these chemicals over time are especially concerning to me. As such, I am a strong proponent of choosing organic dairy products, at least for the dairy foods that are consumed very regularly. Skim milk and plain yogurt are often consumed staples in my household so I only purchase organic varieties.

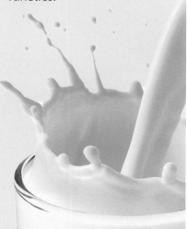

CANNED GOODS

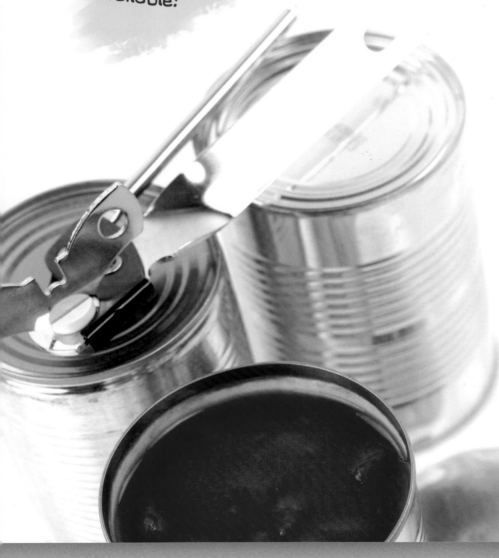

Always choose reduced sodium varieties when available!

Let's Go Shopping For Canned Goods!

Although canned goods offer convenience and value, with a few notable exceptions, they are nutritionally inferior to their "fresh" or "frozen" counterparts. Because of the high temperatures used in the canning process, heat-sensitive nutrients like vitamin C and B vitamins can be significantly diminished. Additionally, most canned vegetables contain excessive sodium while many canned fruits come with extra sugar. Lastly, canned goods can boost exposure to BPA. BPA or bisphenol A is a chemical used to make various plastics including those that line most canned goods. There are growing health concerns in regards to BPA exposures, especially for a developing fetus and young children.

Ground Rules

➤ Recognize that canned goods, with the exceptions that follow, are generally less nutritious than fresh or frozen.

➤ Choose the canned goods that retain excellent nutritional value and have lots to offer: any form of tomato product, any form of beans, 100% pumpkin, 100% sweet potato puree, and canned seafood products. I consider every one of these canned foods superstars!

➤ Always choose reduced sodium varieties when available.

Shopping List
Canned Goods

✓ Any form of canned or bottled tomato product— whole, crushed, diced, sauce, paste, marinara

✓ Any variety of beans or peas—black beans, kidney beans, pinto beans, crowder peas, field peas, navy beans, chic peas, white beans, etc. (there are many others)

✓ 100% pumpkin (not "pie filling")

✓ 100% sweet potato puree (not "pie filling")

✓ Canned broths

✓ Broth and tomato-based soups (not the cream-based varieties)

✓ Olives, pickles, capers, water chestnuts, artichoke hearts, roasted red peppers, pimentos

✓ Canned salmon (red is better than pink), canned tuna (chunk lite has the least mercury and is best for children and women of childbearing ages), sardines, oysters, clams

GRAINS & CEREAL

Reach For Lentils

Like their bean cousins, lentils are cheap, versatile, filling and power-packed with fiber, protein, key minerals, B-vitamins and antioxidants. They provide more folate than any other food and have an edge over the other dried legumes because they cook quickly, require no pre-soaking, and for many, cause less gas.

Let's Go Shopping For Grains!

To me, the "most improved" sections of the grocery store in terms of healthy choices can be found in the aisles housing grain-based foods. Thanks to the flood of new science trumpeting the awesome goodness whole grains offer, this superior starch is in the midst of a renaissance. Never before have there been so many wholesome 100% whole grain foods available to consumers. That being said, unfortunately those notoriously popular, refined, processed, bad-for-you starches like white flour products, white rice, and sugary cereals are still everywhere, so be careful! Please also note that "fiber-fortified" grain-based foods (typically cereals, cereal bars and breads) may not be as healthy as you perceive. Adding extracted fiber (commonly chicory root) to boost up a food's fiber content has no proven health value. Indeed, only fiber that is naturally found in foods by the hand of Mother Nature—like that in physically-intact whole grains and beans—has the science to back it up!

Ground Rules

➤ **Only choose 100% whole grain products.** Thankfully, you can now find virtually every grain-based food desired in this form. Look for "100% whole wheat" or "100% whole grain" on the label or package.

➤ **Recognize that physically intact whole grains like oatmeal and brown rice are a healthier choice than whole grain or whole wheat bread or flour-based products.**

➤ **Do not be duped by grain-based foods that say "contains whole grains" or "made with whole grains."** These phrases are a dead-ringer give away that the product is not 100% whole grain and is usually an unhealthy choice.

Let's Go Shopping For Cereal!

There is generally an entire aisle devoted to this popular breakfast food, so I want to clear up any confusion you have and make sure you know exactly how to make a healthy choice. The right breakfast cereals offer one of the easiest and most convenient ways to fully exploit the wonderful health rewards whole grains offer.

Ground Rules

➤ **Make sure all of your cereal choices are 100% whole grain.** Look for "100%" on the label or the word "whole" before any grains listed in the ingredients list.

➤ **For all selections**—refer to the "nutritional facts" box and be sure it lists five grams or more of fiber per serving and 10 grams or less of sugar per serving. (For young children, three grams of fiber is acceptable, but not for you!)

SHOPPING LIST

GRAINS

✓ Physically intact grains:
  » Plain oatmeal (not flavored)—steel cut or old-fashioned are best
  » Brown rice, black rice, wild rice
  » Barley, quinoa, wheat berries, farro, amaranth, triticale, millet, buckwheat

✓ Wheat germ, oat bran

✓ 100% whole wheat or 100% whole grain bread products—sliced bread, pita breads, bagels, English Muffins, hamburger buns, deli flats. Do not buy unless you see 100% on the label!

✓ 100% whole grain or whole wheat bread alternatives—wraps, tortillas, flat breads. Again, you must see 100% on the label!

✓ 100% whole wheat pasta varieties

✓ Multigrain pasta varieties—many brands available, but I find Barilla Plus brand (yellow box) to have the very best texture and flavor. It will pass for white pasta for practically everyone

✓ Dried beans, peas, lentils—any variety

✓ Plain grits—stone ground is best

✓ 100% whole wheat pizza crust—Mama Mary's and Boboli are two available brands.

✓ Whole wheat flour, whole grain flour, whole grain cornmeal—for baking needs.

> There are many selections that satisfy the ground rules. Here is a list of good choices. (Note - this is not a comprehensive list. Feel free to select any brand that satisfies the ground rules noted above.)

CEREALS

✓ Quaker: Oat Bran, Oat Squares or Old Fashioned Oats

✓ Uncle Sam Original

✓ Nature's Path: Flax Plus, Optimum, Heritage

✓ Kashi: Autumn Wheat, Cinnamon Harvest, Go Lean Crisp, Heart-to-Heart, Go Lean

✓ Kelloggs: Wheat Chex, Multi-Bran Chex, Special K Low-fat Granola, Special K Protein Plus, All-bran, Bran Flakes, Frosted Mini-Wheats

✓ Post: Plain Shredded Wheat, Grape Nuts, Bran Flakes, Great Grains

✓ John McCanns Steel Cut Irish Oatmeal or Old Fashioned Oats

✓ Kretschmer Wheat Germ or Oat Bran (great for topping cereals or adding to smoothies)

*Note many others are available that fit my guidelines.

Don't Forget The...
BAKERY

Most all grocers now offer "fresh baked" goods that are particularly alluring. Whether it is the irresistible smell of fresh-baked bread or the free samples of the day's featured "sweet," the bakery section seems to pull most of us in. Unfortunately, the bakery section has very few healthy options and loads of unhealthy ones. Although some of the fresh baked breads contain some whole grains, most of the offerings are not worthy of being on my shopping list.

Ground Rules

✓ Choose fresh baked breads that contain generous amounts of whole grains. Look for those providing at least two grams of fiber per ounce and be sure the first ingredient in the ingredients list is "whole wheat flour!" Unfortunately 100% whole wheat or 100% whole grain fresh-baked products are very rare in the bakery section.

✓ Avoid pastries, doughnuts, danish, muffins and sweet rolls. Breakfast should be breakfast, not dessert.

✓ Avoid all refined flour (white flour) bread products—bagels, biscuits, buns, bread, etc. Note—the first ingredient in the ingredients list will be "enriched wheat flour," which is white flour.

OILS & CONDIMENTS

Let's Go Shopping For Cooking Oils!

I am equally as passionate about eating for pleasure as I am eating for maximizing my health, so I am particularly grateful for the cooking oil section of the supermarket. Fat is what gives our foods flavor, and if you know exactly which oils to select, you get the best of both worlds—great tasting food that guards and protects your health too. Remember, it is the type of fat in your diet that really matters. Your goals are to bring in the make-me-healthier fats (monounsaturated and omega 3 fats) and to keep the unhealthy fats (saturated and trans fats) out.

Ground Rules

➤ **Make extra virgin olive oil (a monounsaturated fat) your oil of choice.**

➤ **Select canola oil (a monounsaturated fat) for baking and for food preparations where the strong flavor of olive oil is not desired.** "High heat" (check labels) varieties are best for cooking/baking.

➤ **Choose peanut oil, sesame oil, grape seed oil, or coconut oil for very high heat (pan-frying, stir frying, etc.).**

➤ **Use specialty nut oils as needed in recipes**—walnut oil, macadamia oil, etc.

➤ **Use pan/cooking sprays when you want less fat and to keep foods from sticking to pots and pans.**

➤ **Avoid the oils high in omega 6 fats (Americans consume too much of this fat)**—corn oil, soybean oil (also called "vegetable oil"), safflower oil and sunflower oil.

➤ **Strictly avoid all shortenings like Crisco.**

Dr. Ann's Tip
FOR SELECTING OILS

All oils are uniquely susceptible to oxidation, which can diminish their nutritional benefits and their flavor. Oxidation of oils is accelerated by heat, light, and exposure to air. To maximize the flavor and healthfulness of your oils, buy them in small quantities (i.e. turn them over quickly) and store them in the refrigerator. The exception is olive oil, which will solidify in the fridge, making it difficult for ready use. It is best to keep olive oil in a cool, dark cupboard.

Let's Go Shopping For Condiments!

Strategic use of the right condiments and flavor enhancers offers a delicious opportunity to boost both the healthfulness and the flavor of your foods and dishes. I encourage you to get into the habit of using the right ones regularly.

Ground Rules

➤ **Choose reduced sodium varieties when available.**

➤ **Store-bought salad dressing will never be as tasty and healthy as those you can make at home.** I strongly recommend that you make your own and know from experience that you can do it in less than three minutes. If you insist on buying them:

• Choose olive oil or canola oil-based vinaigrettes as your top choice.

• Light or reduced fat salad dressings are also acceptable. Avoid the full fat, thicker varieties like ranch, blue cheese, thousand island, etc. (a little bit does not go a long way) and fat-free dressings have too much sugar.

➤ **Avoid bottled fat-based sauces like alfredo.**

SHOPPING LIST

✓ Extra virgin olive oil

✓ Canola oil ("high heat" best for cooking/ baking)

✓ Peanut oil, sesame oil, coconut oil (for your "occasional" frying)

✓ Pan/cooking sprays – olive oil or canola oil based best for low to moderate heat, refined grape seed or coconut oil based best for high heat

✓ Specialty nut oils – walnut oil, macadamia oil, hazelnut oil etc. (as needed for recipes)

✓ Vinegar – any variety

✓ Sauces – Ketchup, light mayo, olive oil or canola-based regular mayo, mustards, hot sauce, light teriyaki, horseradish, light soy sauce, steak sauce, Worcestershire sauce, pesto, tomato based pasta sauces

✓ Peanut butter (any variety acceptable, but natural varieties best), almond butter, tahini

✓ Flax seeds, chia seeds, hemp seeds

✓ Pure cocoa powder

✓ Any dried herbs or spices (Use liberally as they are filled with remarkably beneficial plant compounds.)

✓ Sundried tomatoes

✓ 100% maple syrup, honey, black strap molasses (use these "natural" sweeteners in moderation)

✓ 100% fruit spreads (berry-based best) like Polaner Fancy Fruit with Fiber or Smuckers Simply Fruit brands. (fruit spreads superior to most jellies and jams)

✓ Salad dressings – If homemade is not an option, choose vinaigrettes that are made with canola and/or olive oil. (Check ingredients list) Regular or reduced fat/lite.

Choosing The Best...
EXTRA VIRGIN OLIVE OIL

I am an admitted foodie that is obsessed with the wonderful flavor of high quality extra virgin olive oil and equally intrigued by its unique healthy profile. The term "extra virgin" signifies that the oil has been "cold pressed" from freshly picked olives (think of it as fresh squeezed olive juice) and it is filled with a remarkable array of potent antioxidant and anti-inflammatory compounds (200 plus) along with healthy monounsaturated fats. Unfortunately, many commercial extra virgin olive oils, especially the Italian brands, may not be pure, freshly squeezed olive oil (likely upwards of 50 percent). These imposters are diluted, adulterated, and manufactured in ways that significantly reduce the healthful properties we desire.

If you want to know you are getting the real McCoy, seek out a specialty olive oil boutique that allows you to taste test the various extra virgin olive oils. If a specialty store is not available, you can order "certified extra virgin olive oil" online from California. These Californian grown and produced oils have been subjected to very rigorous quality standards from the California Olive Oil Council and are guaranteed to be "extra virgin." This is my preferred source. You can learn more and find out where to order at **www.cooc.com**. If you buy your extra virgin olive oil from the standard supermarkets, be sure to select those that come in dark glass bottles. Ideally, the harvest date should be printed on the label. These features boost the chances of authenticity.

DELI

Let's Go Shopping For Deli Products!

The right deli meats and cheeses are delicious, super convenient and can help you build a sandwich or entrée salad that can stack up to the healthiest lunch.

Ground Rules

➤ **Choose deli cheeses that are lower in calories and fat. Ask for "reduced fat" options.** If reduced fat options are not available, lacey Swiss, provolone and mozzarella will usually be the healthiest choices.

➤ **Choose nitrate/nitrite free, lean deli meats—roast beef, turkey and chicken.** Boar's Head, Dietz-Watson, and Applegate Farms brands have an abundance of nitrate free selections. Check labels.

➤ **Take advantage of the convenient rotisserie turkey breasts and whole chickens.**

➤ **Avoid all processed varieties of luncheon meats**—ham, bolognas, wursts, sausages, franks, and loaves.

➤ **Always choose reduced or lower sodium options for meats and cheeses if available.**

➤ **Reserve artisan cheeses for special occasions or as an occasional treat.**

Beware Of The...
DANGER ZONE

Food safety experts have determined that potentially harmful bacteria can multiply rapidly in any perishable food left between 40° and 140° F for more than two hours. This 40–140 temperature range has this been aptly labeled the "Danger Zone." To avoid food borne illness, be sure to keep cold foods below 40° F and hot foods above 140° F!

Shopping List

Deli

✓ Nitrate/nitrite free deli turkey, chicken, or roast beef. Reduced sodium is best.

✓ Deli cheeses—reduced fat/reduced sodium is best.

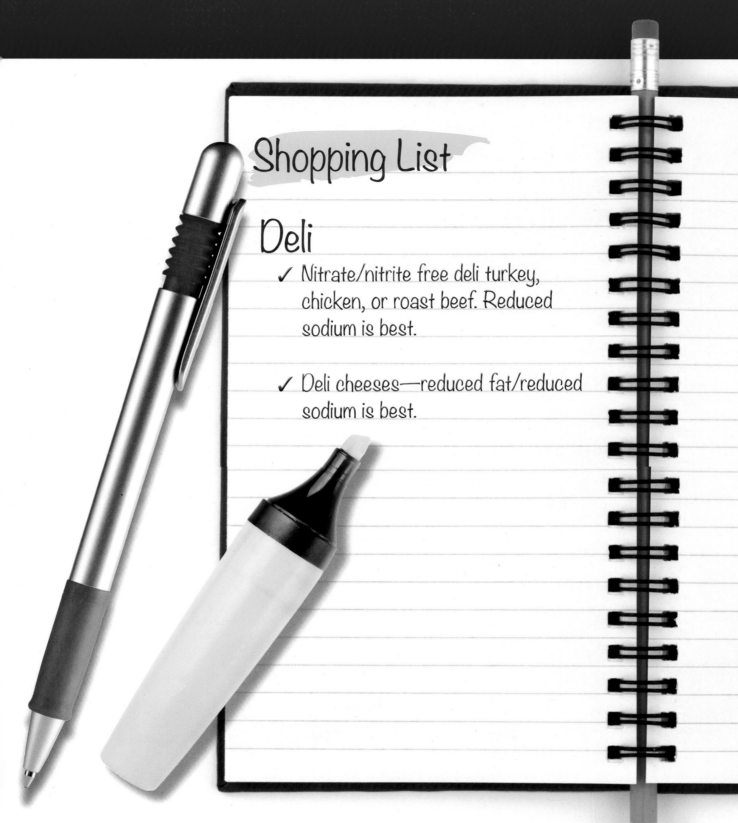

SNACKS

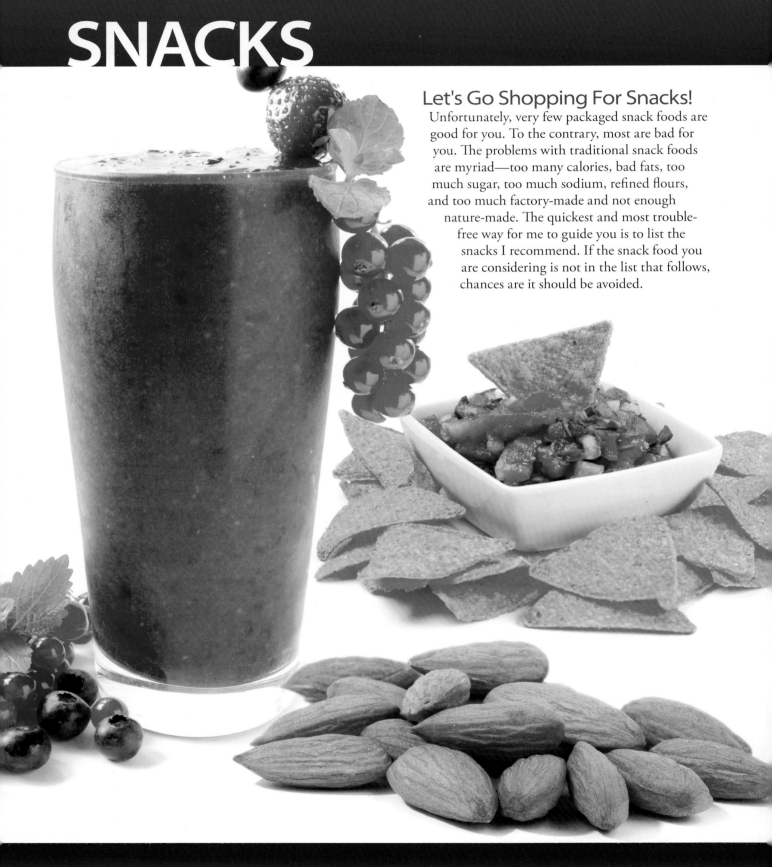

Let's Go Shopping For Snacks!

Unfortunately, very few packaged snack foods are good for you. To the contrary, most are bad for you. The problems with traditional snack foods are myriad—too many calories, bad fats, too much sugar, too much sodium, refined flours, and too much factory-made and not enough nature-made. The quickest and most trouble-free way for me to guide you is to list the snacks I recommend. If the snack food you are considering is not in the list that follows, chances are it should be avoided.

Snacks

✓ Nuts/Seeds—any variety, packaged or bulk, raw or roasted (a handful of nuts is my top rated snack).

✓ Cut fresh veggies (carrots, celery, bell peppers, broccoli, cauliflower)—dip in hummus/bean dips, guacamole, salsa, or olive oil and vinegar.

✓ Fresh or frozen fruit.

✓ Soy nuts, dried wasabi peas.

✓ Whole grain crackers (Wasa, Ak-mak, Triscuits, Kashi Heart to Heart, Multigrain Wheat Thins, Ryvita, Brown rice cakes) with cheese, peanut butter, hummus, salsa, guacamole, sardines, smoked salmon.

✓ "Healthy" chips—R.W. Garcia Tortilla Chips, Terra Vegetable Chips, Food Should Taste Good Tortilla Chips, Sun Chips.

✓ Low fat plain yogurt (sweeten with fresh fruit or a little maple syrup, molasses, or spreadable fruit if you must).

✓ Part-skim mozzarella or other reduced fat (2% milk) cheeses (try convenient cheese sticks).

✓ Homemade fruit smoothies, unsweetened apple sauce.

✓ Dried fruit (avoid if overweight/diabetic)—apricots, apples, peaches, raisins, and plums have the least sugar.

✓ Dried 100% whole grain cereals.

✓ Kashi Granola bars, trail mix.

✓ Hard-boiled omega 3 eggs.

✓ Dark chocolate—70% or more cacao (in moderation).

TRANS FATS

Where Trans Fats Hide In The Grocery Store

Thanks to new labeling regulations passed in 2006, those terribly unhealthy trans fats have made a rapid exodus from the American food supply. But their departure has not been 100 percent, and sadly, they are still lurking in some processed foods.

Based on my most recent scrutiny of food labels, this man-made toxic form of fat still hides in many of the following food items: frozen pizza, cookies, pie crusts, microwave popcorn, stick margarine, cake mixes and frostings, pancake and waffle mixes, frozen dinners, refrigerated and frozen desserts, refrigerated biscuit and pastry dough, and frozen breaded fish and chicken products.

If you plan to purchase any of these foods, be sure to scan its nutritional facts box for "trans fats," and get rid of it quick if any number other than "0" is listed!

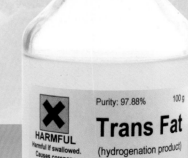

FROZEN

Dr. Ann's Frozen Food Tips

Always be on the lookout for your favorite frozen foods that go on special. When they do—stock up. I eat loads of frozen organic chopped spinach and will buy up to ten bags at a time when it goes on sale.

Let's Go Shopping For Frozen Foods!

First and foremost, recognize that the right frozen foods are just as nutritious as their fresh alternatives. The name of the game in the frozen food section is being vigilant in selecting whole, real, nature-made foods and turning a blind eye to the ever-growing empire of prepared-for-you, packaged, processed foods. Ignore them all (isn't that liberating!). For most, they are quintessential industrial-made food-like offerings and not real food. To see for yourself—check out the ingredients list on a typical frozen dinner package. When chemical terms outnumber recognizable foods ingredients, it is no longer real food in my book!

Ground Rules

➤ **Select whole, real foods only. All frozen foods will have an ingredients list on the package.** To be a wholesome selection, there should be very few ingredients listed.

➤ **Don't even consider the frozen "prepared" foods**—forget the side dishes, entrees, and of course the frozen dinners. This makes getting through the frozen food aisles so easy and so quick!

➤ **Avoid frozen veggies with added butter or sauces.**

➤ **Avoid frozen fruits with added sugars.**

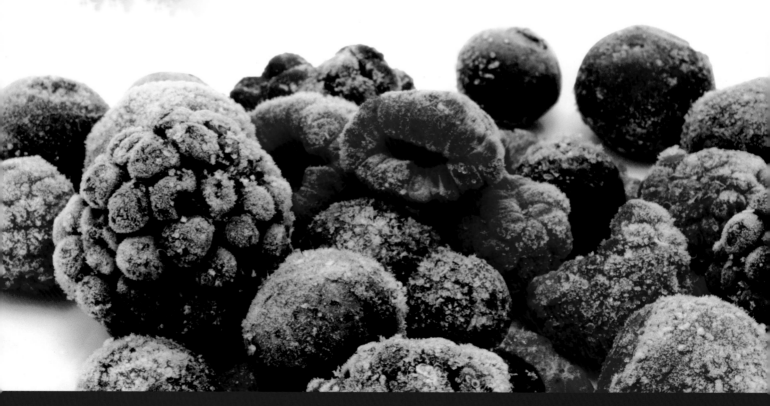

Shopping List

✓ Frozen vegetables—any variety (no added butter/sauces)

✓ Frozen fruits—any variety (no added sugars)

✓ Frozen seafood—plain fish, shrimp, scallops, mussels, crab (nothing breaded or fried)

✓ Frozen poultry—plain chicken or turkey. Skinless boneless chicken breasts and tenderloins are super convenient. (nothing breaded or fried)

✓ Frozen whole grain products—waffles (Kashi brand is good), bread (Ezekiel 4:9 brand is excellent)

✓ Frozen desserts—100% fruit sorbets, reduced fat/lite ice creams and yogurt blends as an occasional (not regular) treat. Breyers Smooth and Dreamy, Edy's Slow Churned Light, Dreyer's Slow Churned Light and Purely Decadent Coconut Milk vanilla ice cream are healthier choices.

FROZEN

I love the convenience of frozen (unseasoned) cut vegetable medleys for an instant lunch or dinner stir-fry. Many appetizing blends are now available, including Asian and Mediterranean.

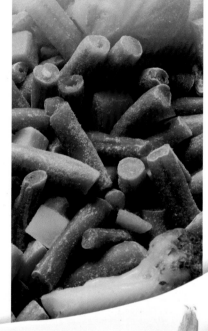

BEVERAGES

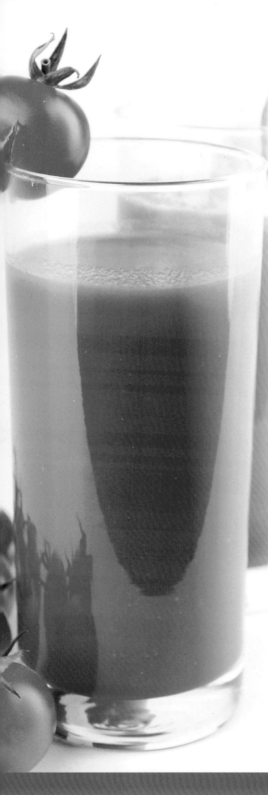

Let's Go Shopping For Beverages!

We are going to make this one really easy. With rare exceptions, my advice for making healthy beverage selections in the grocery store (largely an oxymoron) is to avoid them all. Yes, I am directing you to completely ignore the entire aisle of bottled sodas, waters, fruit drinks, teas, coffees and other specialty beverages. My reasons are just as straightforward. First, these ever-popular beverages offer zero to minimal nutrients and in the case of sugary ones, which make up the majority—they are filled with rapidly absorbable sugars that have emerged as the most fattening and metabolically stressful form of calories on the planet. And for those you may think are "healthy," like the fitness and vitamin waters or bottled green teas, do not be duped. Many contain sugars just like soda and there is no evidence that they have any true health value.

Ground Rules

➤ **Strictly avoid any type of sugary beverages**—soda, fruit drinks, teas, coffees, and vitamin/fitness waters.

➤ **Avoid artificially sweetened beverages**—sodas, flavored waters, teas, and fruit drinks. Although they may be a better choice than sugary beverages, they are not in any way healthy.

➤ **Restrict the use of sports beverages for situations involving vigorous physical activity and sweating (especially those exceeding one hour).** Prior to physical activity and within the first one-hour, water is the healthiest hydrator.

➤ **Recognize that tap water is infinitely cheaper and more rigorously tested and monitored than bottled water.** Reserve bottled waters for situations where tap water is unavailable, the taste of the tap water is unacceptable to you, or if you have safety concerns about the available tap water supply.

➤ **Recognize that 100% fruit juices are a concentrated source of sugars and calories, and that it is always better to eat your fruit than drink it.**

Where Does Your
CITY RANK?

If you live in a city with a population greater than 250,000, check out where your city's water supply ranks in the Environmental Working Group's (EWG) Big City Water Rankings. At EWG, a team of experts performs comprehensive reviews of government reports, scientific studies, and its own laboratory tests to determine the safety of municipal water supplies. Find out more at **EWG.org/tap-water/rating-big-city-water/**.

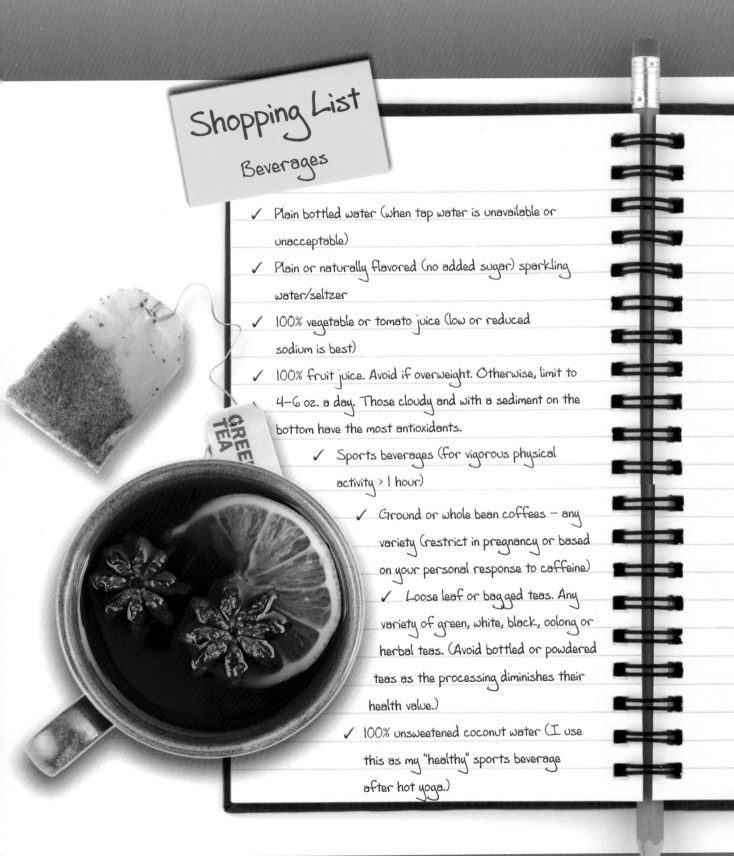

Shopping List
Beverages

✓ Plain bottled water (when tap water is unavailable or unacceptable)

✓ Plain or naturally flavored (no added sugar) sparkling water/seltzer

✓ 100% vegetable or tomato juice (low or reduced sodium is best)

✓ 100% fruit juice. Avoid if overweight. Otherwise, limit to 4–6 oz. a day. Those cloudy and with a sediment on the bottom have the most antioxidants.

✓ Sports beverages (for vigorous physical activity > 1 hour)

✓ Ground or whole bean coffees — any variety (restrict in pregnancy or based on your personal response to caffeine)

✓ Loose leaf or bagged teas. Any variety of green, white, black, oolong or herbal teas. (Avoid bottled or powdered teas as the processing diminishes their health value.)

✓ 100% unsweetened coconut water (I use this as my "healthy" sports beverage after hot yoga.)

Dining Out… Healthy And Happy

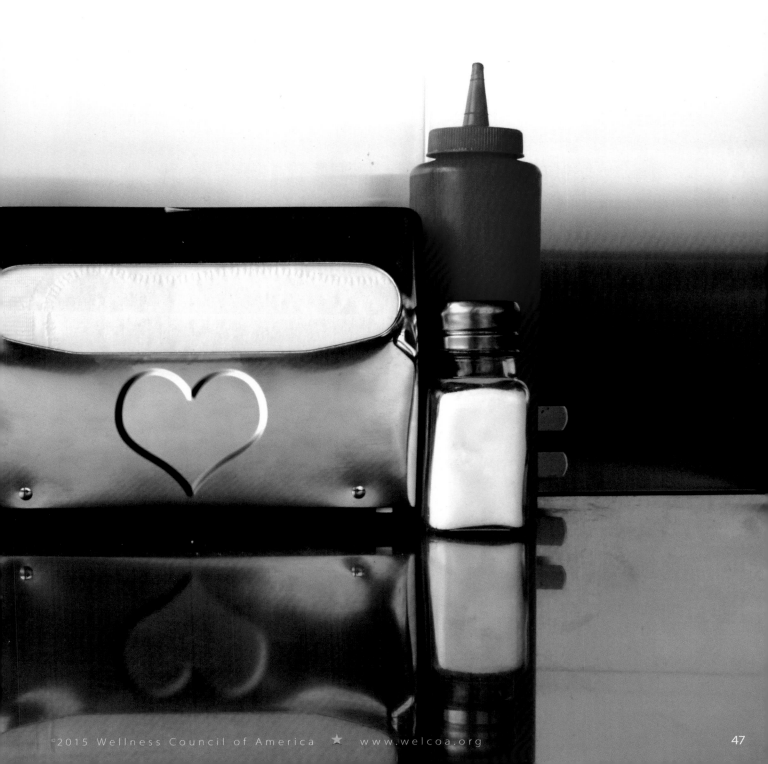

Dining Out… Healthy <u>And</u> Happy

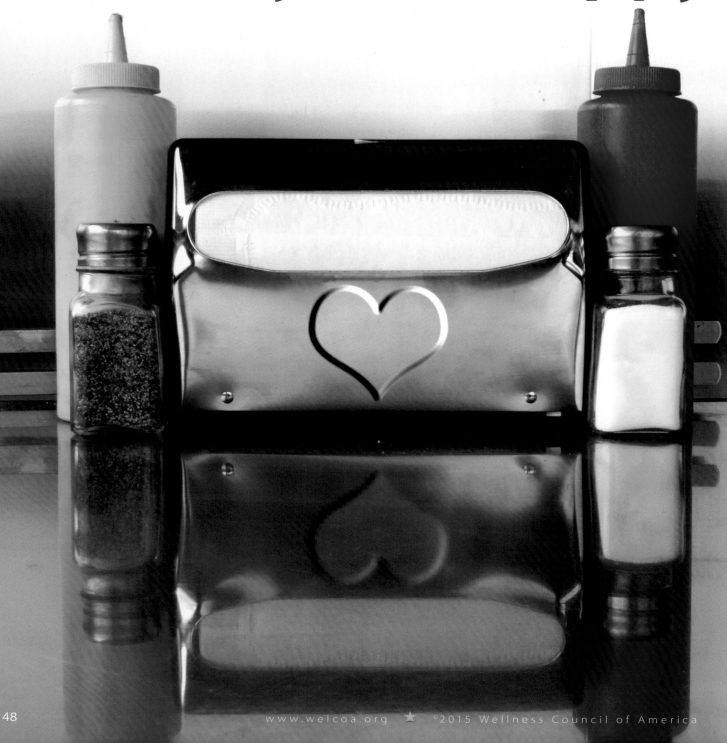

Now, we are going to totally switch course and conquer healthy eating away from home. I am especially excited to guide you through this leg of our journey because I firmly believe this is where we venture most off track, sometimes profoundly so.

Over the past few decades, *the most dramatic shift* in our dietary habits has been the replacement of home-cooked meals with foods prepared by restaurants, especially fast food restaurants. Not long ago, dining out was reserved for special occasions like graduations, birthdays, and anniversaries, but for many Americans, it is now a routine part of daily living. The average American consumes three burgers and four orders of fries a week from outside the home! With over 560,000 dining establishments available to feed us, many of which market their fare incessantly, it is no wonder that we now spend about 50% of our food budgets (up from 25% in 1970) and consume up to 40% of our calories from meals prepared by others.

Epic changes in our external nutritional environment are at the root of this striking swing from eating home-prepared foods to restaurant foods. The most notable difference has been the relentless onslaught of fast foods. This intensely high-risk fare is now everywhere. The number of fast food spots has more than doubled since the '70s, out-pacing any other type of restaurant. Nowadays, you can readily get fast food in schools, gas stations, universities, airports, zoos, parks, trains, sports arenas, Target, Wal-Mart, K-Mart, and even hospitals. The sad truth is that as long as it is there, we will eat it. In 1970, we only spent $6 billion on fast food. This year we will spend over $100 billion on it.

Over the same period of time, rates of diet-related chronic diseases including obesity, type 2 diabetes and metabolic syndrome have skyrocketed. Record numbers of Americans have lost their health, and healthcare spending has reached unimaginable levels that threaten our continued existence as a strong and prosperous nation. I believe, with every thread of my body, that the biggest culprit is our reliance on others to provide our meals and the notoriously poor choices we tend to make in this context.

Fortunately, there is some good news, too—just like in the grocery store, healthy, wholesome, good-for-you options have never been more plentiful in the outside food world. I know because I've made about twenty-five business trips this past year and spent many weekends over the last ten on the road, while traveling to my kid's sports competitions. And when it comes to practicing what I preach, I don't just walk my talk, I run it! If I can readily triumph nutritionally in our big, scary, largely toxic restaurant food culture, I know you can too!

In the pages that follow, I am going to share every ounce of healthy dining wisdom I have accumulated during my frequent forays into the real world. Just like my grocery clinic, my guidance promises to be direct, concise, and 100 percent candid. I am certain the information that follows can improve your health and vitality, and perhaps even save your life, so it is my greatest hope that you will take it to heart, mind, and body. For now, take a deep, invigorating breath, and get ready to learn exactly how to not only survive, but also thrive in our modern food culture.

Dining Out Means…
MORE CALORIES!

There is widespread scientific consensus that dining out increases the risk of eating excess calories and well-conducted studies confirm it. According to a comprehensive evaluation by USDA researchers, here is what you can expect in terms of extra calories when you choose to eat foods away from home.

➤ Each additional meal or snack consumed outside of the home comes with an average of 134 extra calories versus the same meals or snacks prepared at home. (Keep in mind that if you did this just once a day with no increase in exercise, over the course of one year you would gain an additional 15 pounds!)

➤ For the average adult, eating out for lunch has the greatest impact, boosting daily calories by 158. Having dinner away from home adds an additional 144 calories; breakfast 74 calories; and snacks 100 calories.

➤ Overweight individuals are at the greatest risk of consuming extra calories when eating away from home. For a person with a body mass index (BMI) in the obese range (≥30), dining out adds an additional 239 daily calories.

Why Dining Out Is Oh-So-Risky For Health And Weight Gain

Before I provide my best guidance for dining out, I want to make sure you have a firm grasp on the underlying forces and features of the restaurant world that can trip us up and derail our health. As I already professed, I firmly believe that the vast and frequent consumption of restaurant-based foods, especially fast foods, which has come to define dining in the new millennium, has completely wrecked our health. There are a host of common features in restaurant foods that make them particularly perilous, and I want you to be fully aware of each and how they ultimately do their dirty work. In fact, I suggest that you read this section multiple times.

Big Portions. As humans, we are hard-wired to consume the entirety of the foods served to us. This is a firmly documented, innate behavioral trait common to all humans, and likely stems from the famine and starvation our ancient ancestors often faced. Yes, we are instinctively inclined to eat all the food in our midst by nature. Unfortunately, over the past three decades there has been an enormous increase in the standard serving sizes of foods offered in restaurants, and of course, we are eating it. According to scientists, for every restaurant-based food they have examined, the portion size has significantly increased over the past 30 years. In fact, if you clean your plate today, you are consuming an average of 50% more calories than you would have in the 1960s. Over this time span, burgers have gone from 1.5 ounces up to 8 ounces; fries have gone from 2.4 ounces up to 7.1 ounces; sodas have gone from 6.5 ounces up to 42 ounces; pasta entrees have gone from 1.5 cups to 3 cups; muffins have gone from 2-3 ounces to 5-7 ounces; and you can find cookies the size of serving platters in the mall! Knowing that it is a deeply entrenched facet of human nature to eat all of the food we are given, it doesn't take a weight loss expert to grasp the OVERWHELMING influence portion sizes have on the weight that stares back at you when you step onto the bathroom scale.

High Glycemic Load Carbohydrates. The glycemic load of a carb food signifies how fast and how high blood glucose levels rise after you consume it. The greater a food's glycemic load, the quicker and the higher your blood sugar level climbs and the worse it is for your body weight, your arteries, and your metabolic health. Diets with a high glycemic load have been linked to weight gain, heart disease, type 2 diabetes, metabolic syndrome, and some cancers. Restaurants are notorious on the glycemic front because of the hefty load of refined, low-fiber, easy-to-digest carbohydrates so widespread on their menus. White potatoes, white rice, sweets, sugary beverages, and white flour-based products like hamburger buns, biscuits, bagels, muffins, rolls, breads, pastries, pasta, and pizza make up the list of the highest glycemic load foods and are, by far, the most plentiful carb offerings. These foods, especially in standard (i.e. oversized) restaurant portions, will do a doozy on your blood sugar.

High Caloric Density. The greater the number of calories in a given volume of food, the higher its caloric density and the more fattening it tends to be. Foods with a high caloric density provide a 1-2 punch for weight gain. First, compact packages of calories make it quicker and easier to consume excessive amounts of them (they go down fast and easy) and secondly, they do not offer the appetite-suppressing power of volume. Believe it or not, when it comes to suppressing the human appetite—volume trumps calories. In other words, our bodies desire a certain volume of food first and foremost versus a certain number of calories. And unfortunately, we will be primed to keep eating until our food volume needs are satisfied. Foods with the highest energy density (lots of calories in small amounts) are those high in fat and low in water, and fiber. Sadly, the most popular menu options in fast food and casual dining chains fit this very description including burgers, hot dogs, french fries, pizza, fried chicken, fried seafood, pasta with cream sauces, biscuits, nachos, and anything else smothered in cheese.

Excess Sodium. Currently, 88 percent of Americans exceed the recommended intake of dietary sodium (2,300 mg/day). For high risk populations, including those over 50, African Americans, and those with high blood pressure, diabetes, or kidney disease—a whopping 99 percent consume more than the recommended 1,500 mg a day. Consuming too much sodium increases the risk of heart attacks, strokes, high blood pressure, osteoporosis, gastric cancer and kidney disease. The truth is that we cannot just blame the saltshaker for our sodium-laden diets. Seventy-five percent of the sodium in our diets comes from packaged, manufactured foods and foods served in restaurants. It is nearly impossible to dine out in most chain restaurants and not surpass your recommended daily sodium intake. A typical value-sized meal of a burger and fries provides up to 2,500 mg of sodium. A single bacon cheeseburger can top out at 2,400 mg of sodium. That is what I would call a sodium grenade!

Ultra Palatable Foods. As humans, our taste buds have a highly developed and powerful affinity for fat, salt, and sugar. Combine any two, or

Dear Brain,

Please cut this burger in two and eat only one of the halves now. Then, take the rest home, save it for lunch tomorrow and I will love you for life!

Love,

Your Heart

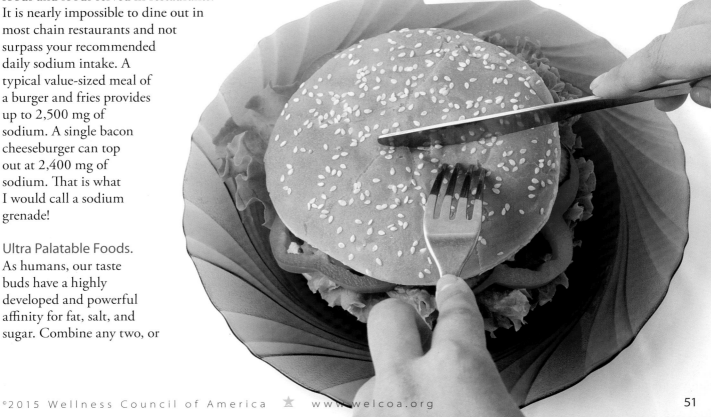

More Fast Food =
MORE OBESITY

In a recent study that examined the relationship between the numbers of fast food outlets per capita relative to rates of obesity in 26 wealthy nations, scientists uncovered some stunning associations. The US had the highest concentration of fast food restaurants (7.52 per 100,000 people) and the highest rates of obesity (31.3 percent for men and 33.2 percent for women). In striking contrast, Norway and Japan had much lower fast food densities (.13 to .19 per 100,000 people, respectively) and much lower obesity rates—for Japan, 2.5 percent (men) and 3.3 percent (women), and for Norway, 6.4 percent (men) and 5.9 percent (women).

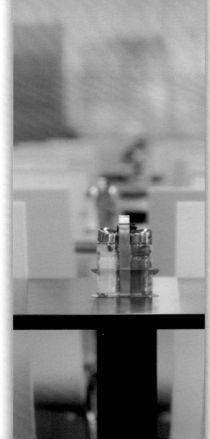

better yet all three in the same food or meal, and the gustatory response is true bliss—both in the mouth and the brain. In terms of appetite control (which is the Holy Grail for weight control), one of the most important and provocative scientific advancements of the past decade has been a new understanding of how the flavor profile of specific foods impacts our appetite at the level of the brain. A quickly mounting body of medical research is showing that highly flavorful, super-palatable foods (the ones high in fat, salt and/or sugar) can rewire and alter the landscape of our brains in such a way that we simply cannot resist eating them. I wish it were not true, but it appears that simply tasting foods rich in fat and or sugar, like cheesecake and chili cheese fries, can directly stimulate the pleasure centers of our brains in the same manner as addictive drugs like morphine or cocaine. Once stimulated, these reward centers then release endorphins (the brain's "feel good" neurochemicals) that provide a blissful, yet transient feeling of great pleasure. Naturally, we want to experience this feeling again, and the consequence can be food addiction. Research in animals and growing research in humans shows that the reward centers of the brain are activated by fatty and sugary foods, and we will go to great lengths in our attempts to secure another food high. It seems the sugar and fat in ultra-palatable foods that are so ubiquitous in restaurants are "reinforcing" and can literally reroute our brain circuits into a vicious, self-perpetuating cycle of overconsumption. Please note that this is something beyond our conscious control. For me, this scenario is the single most frightening risk of dining out on the wrong foods, especially traditional fast foods, with any regularity. In all honesty, this terrifies me and is the number one reason why I NEVER eat traditional fast food, or certain sweets for that matter. Do not underestimate the power of sugary and fatty foods like ice cream, donuts, pastries, cakes, and cookies, along with bacon cheeseburgers, fried chicken, french fries, onion rings, and other classic fast food fare. They will highjack your taste buds, your appetite and your waistline!

Variety. The greater the variety or selection of food choices, the more we tend to order or serve ourselves, and ultimately the more we consume. Behavioral scientists have long observed that food variety stimulates eating behavior. The basis for this behavioral trait likely stems from our dependence on a broad range of essential nutrients distributed amongst a vast array of different foods. Eating a variety of foods would have provided our hunter-gatherer ancestors a better chance of obtaining the full complement of nutrients necessary for survival (and reproduction), and this ancient instinct is locked into our genes. To compound things, variety in food offerings also diminishes our sense of food satisfaction, providing further inducement to eat more. Needless to say, you will find a dizzying menu of options in most all restaurants. In fast food chains, new menu options have even out-paced portion sizes. Traditional burger chains now provide fried chicken, fried fish, wraps, pancakes, biscuits, cinnamon rolls, and the full gamut of other breakfast foods, along with ice cream, smoothies, dessert coffees (up to 80 varieties!), and cookies.

Flavor Variety. Along with food variety, flavor variety also poses hidden challenges. It is well documented that the greater the flavor variety of a food or meal, the more we tend to eat. This reality is due to something called sensory-specific satiety. Housed within our brain's appetite control center of the hypothalamus are areas that respond specifically to distinct flavors or tastes in foods, like sweet, salty, sour, and savory. This means that sweet tastes will stimulate one area, savory another, and so on. When you eat a food, the flavor or flavors within that food will stimulate and awaken the corresponding flavor-specific area or areas within the hypothalamus. Once awakened, each taste-specific area releases the hunger-promoting hormone neuropeptide Y (NPY). When it comes to hunger, NPY can be an enemy to any waistline. The hormone is a particularly powerful appetite stimulator and prompts you to really want food. Turning on multiple areas of the appetite center simultaneously by eating various flavors at once means that the brain will release even more NPY. This leads to more intense appetite stimulation and food-seeking behavior, and ultimately increases the time it takes to feel full.

The food industry, which depends on food consumption for its livelihood, is well aware of this phenomenon and exploits it relentlessly. Almost every item or dish on the menu is a virtual cornucopia of appetite-inciting flavors. With sweet, salty, savory, and sour, along with a spectacular array of newfangled artificial flavors commingling in endless combinations layer upon layer, it's no wonder that we are hungrier than ever— and consuming more than ever!

Diversify Your Diet And Limit The…
FOOD OF THE CORN

One of the most seismic and deleterious shifts in our modern diets has been the profound contraction of dietary diversity. According to paleoanthropologists, our ancient ancestors had access to tens of thousands of edible species of which 3,000 were dietary staples. Today, two-thirds of the calories we consume in America come from just four species—corn, rice, wheat, and soy beans. With corn especially, its iterations of processed forms are endless (think corn oil, high fructose corn syrup, maltodextrin, modified food starch, etc. etc.). In a truly freaky, recent scientific analysis, investigators discovered that corn is an ingredient in nearly every single fast food meal. The research team analyzed 480 servings of fast food burgers, chicken sandwiches, and fries at the atomic level, and found that only 12 of the 480 samples could be traced back to something other than corn. According to the study's author, "Corn is not just a grain used in the production of fast food, it is the basis of all fast food." I urge you to diversify your diet—enough corn is enough!

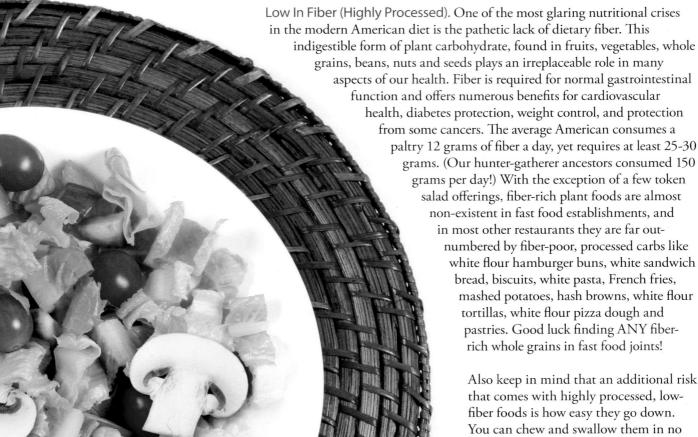

Low In Fiber (Highly Processed). One of the most glaring nutritional crises in the modern American diet is the pathetic lack of dietary fiber. This indigestible form of plant carbohydrate, found in fruits, vegetables, whole grains, beans, nuts and seeds plays an irreplaceable role in many aspects of our health. Fiber is required for normal gastrointestinal function and offers numerous benefits for cardiovascular health, diabetes protection, weight control, and protection from some cancers. The average American consumes a paltry 12 grams of fiber a day, yet requires at least 25-30 grams. (Our hunter-gatherer ancestors consumed 150 grams per day!) With the exception of a few token salad offerings, fiber-rich plant foods are almost non-existent in fast food establishments, and in most other restaurants they are far out-numbered by fiber-poor, processed carbs like white flour hamburger buns, white sandwich bread, biscuits, white pasta, French fries, mashed potatoes, hash browns, white flour tortillas, white flour pizza dough and pastries. Good luck finding ANY fiber-rich whole grains in fast food joints!

Also keep in mind that an additional risk that comes with highly processed, low-fiber foods is how easy they go down. You can chew and swallow them in no time—certainly faster than your body's innate appetite control systems can respond (which is 20-30 minutes). When was the last time you spent 30 minutes eating a burger from a fast food chain?

Excessive Saturated Fats. Saturated fats are the artery clogging "four legged" fats that come from red meat, butter, and whole dairy products like cheese. They are also found in palm oil, a favored fat for deep-frying mediums. Regrettably, these fats are beyond prolific in the world of restaurant foods. Because of the preponderance of bacon, sausage, cheese, cream sauces, burgers, and deep fried foods on menus, it is really tough to keep saturated fat intakes to safe levels when dining out. Cheese is by far the single greatest contributor to the mother lode of saturated fats served up in restaurants. In fact, if you scrutinize the menus in fast food outlets and casual dining chains, you will see that cheese is practically everywhere! The word on the street, within the restaurant industry, is that when it comes to creating tasty fare, smothering anything in cheese always works.

The same goes for bacon. Current dietary recommendations are to limit saturated fats to 7–10% of daily calories. For someone on a 2,000 calorie a day diet, that translates to 16–20 grams a day. If you take a close look at the nutritional facts published for fast food items, you will see many examples of single items, especially those darn bacon cheeseburgers that will put you over your daily limit of saturated fat even without the fries. Appetizers in casual dining chains can be obscenely excessive in saturated fat. Things like cheese fries covered in ranch, smothered nachos, loaded potato skins, and spinach dip appetizers can offer up more than two days worth of saturated fats. And that's even before the entrée. Just writing this makes my heart hurt!

Please be mindful and wary of these harmful, high-risk features found in the restaurant world. They will undoubtedly add to your waistline and take away from your overall health.

Eat More…
WEIGH LESS!

One of the easiest and most powerful strategies for lifelong success with body weight is regularly consuming foods that are big in volume, yet low in calories. And the most effective big, yet waist-whittling foods are none other than fruits and veggies.

The reason is simple physics. The volume of food in your stomach, regardless of calories, has a powerful appetite suppressive effect. Because fruits and vegetables get most of their volume from zero calorie fiber and water, they are the perfect foods for capitalizing on the hunger-quieting power of volume. Likewise, fruits and vegetables are the foods with the lowest energy density. An important study in the *American Journal of Clinical Nutrition* confirmed the effectiveness of this "eat more, weigh less" strategy. In this evaluation, obese study subjects that had the greatest reduction in energy density over a six-month study period (those who ate the most fruits and veggies), lost more than twice as much weight as those with the least reduction in energy density. And this was the case despite the fact that they ate three-quarters of a pound more food a day!

As a double bonus, including more fruits and veggies in your day not only reduces the caloric density of your diet, it also dramatically boosts its nutritional quality. I always include at least one cup of fruit at breakfast and one and one-half cups of veggies at lunch and dinner. If you have not already achieved this milestone in healthy living, I urge you to do so. I know of no other nutritional undertaking that will more quickly transform the way you look and feel while simultaneously turning you into a sound biologic fortress.

With awareness and a solid understanding of the enormous challenges and hazards that come with eating out, I am ready to provide you with my very best personal guidance for the most common dining out experiences. If you adhere to the directives that follow, you can rest assured that you will be making meal selections that are in harmony with good health.

Next time, hold the cheese!

Now, Let's Go Out To Eat—Healthfully!

"Your favorite drive-thru or burger joint actually houses virtually every imaginable feature scientists have identified that one way or another, lead to overeating."

Fast Food Restaurants

Since fast foods now make up the largest share of foods consumed away from home, and because this is where you will typically face the biggest challenges, let's slay that monster first. Just like the beverage aisle in the grocery store, my very best advice is simply these three words, "Don't go there!" I consider traditional fast food places so high risk for weight gain and diet-related maladies like heart attacks and diabetes that the only "best" advice I can give you with a clear conscience is to never step foot in their doors. When I say "traditional," I am referring to the fast food chains that sell burgers, fries, tacos, or fried chicken as their staple selections. Take it from me as someone who never patronizes them, it is profoundly liberating to completely remove the fast food option from your dining out dalliances. No more burgers versus tacos versus fried chicken—talk about simplifying life!

The Perfect Storm

If opting out for easier decision-making doesn't quite do it for you, bear in mind that fast food joints are loaded minefields that make it almost humanly impossible to eat healthy. They really create the "perfect storm" in terms of permitting us to eat too many unhealthy calories with extraordinary ease. Your favorite drive-thru or burger joint actually houses virtually every imaginable feature scientists have identified that one way or another, lead to overeating. And these notorious traits include the following—big portions, high caloric density, high glycemic load, variety in foods and flavors, lack of fiber, convenience, accessibility, and ultra-palatability. Yes, fast food is the most comprehensive embodiment of all the scientifically validated "fattening features" foods could possibly have. Remember too that many of these features affect us in ways totally out of our conscious control.

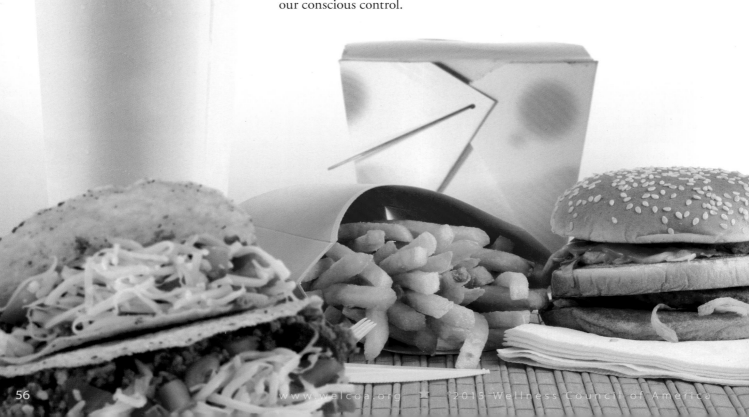

The Science Speaks For Itself

And for those of you who think you do have control—sorry, studies consistently find that even the most aware and disciplined folks will get sucked into the fast food storm. Bottom line—it will always be easier to change your environment (i.e. never go eat there) than to change your mind! And if you are still not convinced that the best fast food is no fast food, I will let the science speak for itself. Here are some scientific highlights regarding how fast food can affect our health.

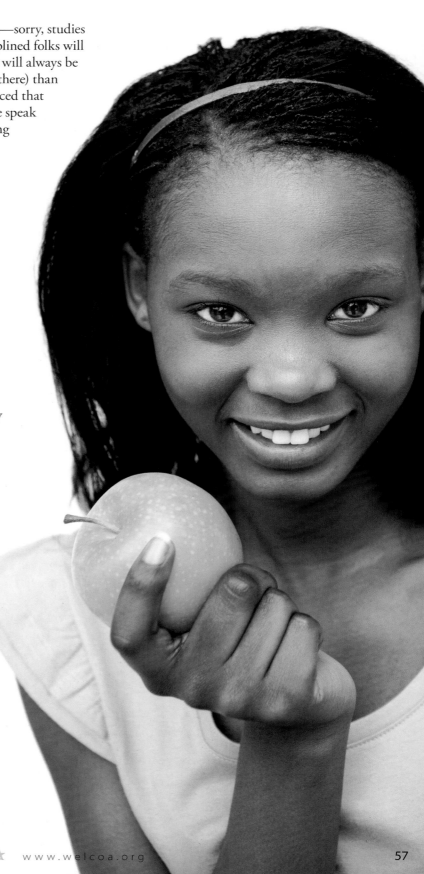

> ➤ In a study involving 3,394 young adults whose dietary habits and weights were monitored over two separate years within a 10-year study period, BMI (body mass index) increased in accordance with the number of fast food meals consumed. For every additional fast food meal eaten weekly, study subjects' weight increased by .9 t o 1.7 pounds over the year.

> ➤ In a study that tracked fast food consumption in 44,072 African American women over a 10 year period, those who ate fast food at least once a week gained more weight and were 40 to 70 percent more likely to develop type 2 diabetes relative to study subjects who never ate fast food.

> ➤ In a landmark study involving 3,000 young adults followed over a 15-year study period, those who consumed fast food more than twice a week gained an additional 10 pounds and increased their risk of obesity by 50 percent. Frequent fast food eaters also doubled their risk of developing insulin resistance (a precursor to type 2 diabetes and other metabolic diseases).

> ➤ After following the dietary habits of 2,379 young girls over a 10 year study period, researchers concluded that the more fast food the girls consumed, the higher their intakes of calories, sodium, and saturated fat.

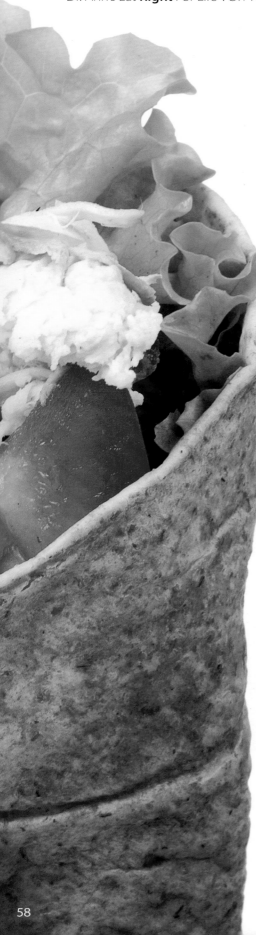

➤ In an analysis of 7,194 adult men and women followed over a median of 28.5 months, those consuming the most "fast foods" specifically burgers, pizza and sausage, gained significantly more weight than those consuming the least.

➤ Each meal consumed in fast food restaurants increases an adolescent's daily caloric intake by 108 calories.

➤ In an evaluation of the nutritional quality of children's meals served in fast food outlets, only three percent met the basic nutritional standards set by the National School Lunch Program.

➤ In a study of more than 9,000 adults, consuming fast food increased the prevalence of overweight by 27–31 percent.

Dr. Ann's…
TRUE CONFESSIONS

I never eat traditional fast food, so I have never had any reason to examine the nutrition information published by fast food outlets for their offerings. While writing this book, however, I scrutinized them closely, and I must admit that I was truly shocked by the nutritional decadence I encountered.

From the mountains of calories, saturated fats, and oh-my-goodness sodium, to the low valleys of refined, fiber-depleted carbs, and the dark crevasses devoid of real food—it really was a jaw-dropping, frightening trek for me, not to mention the daunting peaks of sugar in beverages!

I imagine that many of you reading this book have never taken the journey into fast food nutritional information. I strongly encourage you to do so. Simply Google the name of any fast food chain along with "nutrition PDF"—for example, "McDonald's nutrition PDF" or "Kentucky Fried Chicken nutrition PDF." Every chain has one posted on the web and they are formatted in a manner that makes it easy to quickly view the nutritional profile of each item they offer. Warning: it is a scary trip, but one you need to take to begin your healthy dining journey.

As you travel through the posted nutritional info for a given fast food outlet, keep these "daily (over 24 hours) recommended intakes" for the average adult in mind:

➤ Calories: 2,000 to 2,200

➤ Sodium: <2,300 mg; for high risk individuals < 1,500 mg

➤ Saturated fats: 16 to 22 grams

➤ Added sugars (like in soda): 25 grams for women and 37 grams for men

Because Life Happens

Given the reality that fast food is now everywhere you are, it would be completely unrealistic of me to expect you to totally avoid this inescapable fixture of our modern dining landscape. Lucky for our bodies, there are a growing number of more wholesome and healthy, "contemporary" fast food options out there that I can recommend without a heavy heart.

Abide by the guidelines that follow for the healthiest fast food experience:

➤ Select fast food outlets that have a greater selection of healthy choices. Sandwich and sub-based chains would be my top pick, including places like Subway, Quiznos, Panera Bread, Atlanta Bread, Jason's Deli, and Au Bon Pain. There are certainly bad choices in these establishments, but you can always find the good ones as well. One of the best things about sub chains is that you get to call all of your own nutritional shots. That is the ultimate in environmental food control, so speak up!

✓ Go for sandwiches, subs, or wraps made with whole grain or whole wheat breads. Stay away from white bread and strictly avoid croissants (they are loaded with white flour and fat).

✓ Choose lean protein like deli-sliced turkey, chicken, or roast beef, and avoid processed meats like bacon, ham, corned beef, sausage, meatballs, and cold cuts. Tuna or chicken salad sandwiches are fine if they are made with light or non-fat mayo, which you'll need to inquire.

✓ Ask for every vegetable topping available including lettuce, tomato, onions, olives, peppers, and cucumbers, or go veggie all the way. Do not hesitate to ask for extra veggies. I know from experience that the servers find it refreshing and have never turned me down.

✓ Control your portions. Stick to 6-inch subs. For sandwiches, select the thinnest sliced whole grain bread available (I ask to see the bread options) or remove the top piece of sandwich bread, especially if it is thick-sliced.

✓ Go light on the cheese or hold it completely. Just because they usually put on three slices does not mean you cannot get one or two.

✓ Avoid high fat or high sugar condiments. Mustard, light mayo, a little oil and vinegar, or reduced-fat salad dressings are your best options. Stay away from fat-free sauces and dressings as they are high in sugar.

✓ Season your sandwich or sub liberally with all the available herbs and spices, NOT including salt.

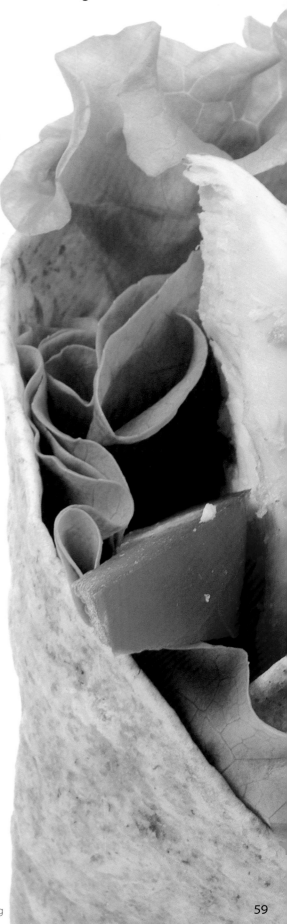

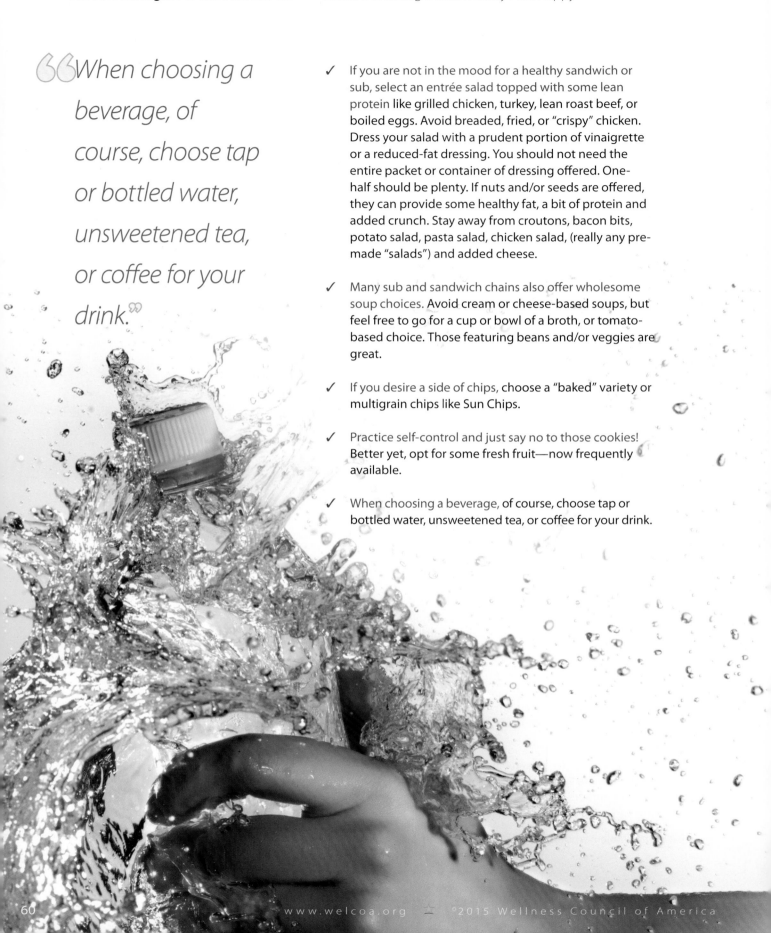

❝When choosing a beverage, of course, choose tap or bottled water, unsweetened tea, or coffee for your drink.❞

✓ If you are not in the mood for a healthy sandwich or sub, select an entrée salad topped with some lean protein like grilled chicken, turkey, lean roast beef, or boiled eggs. Avoid breaded, fried, or "crispy" chicken. Dress your salad with a prudent portion of vinaigrette or a reduced-fat dressing. You should not need the entire packet or container of dressing offered. One-half should be plenty. If nuts and/or seeds are offered, they can provide some healthy fat, a bit of protein and added crunch. Stay away from croutons, bacon bits, potato salad, pasta salad, chicken salad, (really any pre-made "salads") and added cheese.

✓ Many sub and sandwich chains also offer wholesome soup choices. Avoid cream or cheese-based soups, but feel free to go for a cup or bowl of a broth, or tomato-based choice. Those featuring beans and/or veggies are great.

✓ If you desire a side of chips, choose a "baked" variety or multigrain chips like Sun Chips.

✓ Practice self-control and just say no to those cookies! Better yet, opt for some fresh fruit—now frequently available.

✓ When choosing a beverage, of course, choose tap or bottled water, unsweetened tea, or coffee for your drink.

They Made Me Do It!

If somehow you wind up backed into a corner where traditional fast food is absolutely the only option, (which should be extremely rare!) here is my best advice for making the dining experience as damage-free as possible. First and foremost, put up your guard! As I said earlier, even for those with extraordinary self-discipline and self-control—traditional fast food restaurants are filled with a multitude of subtle, yet powerful cues and influences that can push us, and push us hard, to make the wrong choices. This would include the automatic (and obnoxious) verbal prompts from the servers to "value-size" or "super-size."

Commit to the guidelines that follow and give yourself a pat on the back for conquering one of the most difficult of all dietary feats in the modern world—eating healthfully in a traditional fast food restaurant.

General Rules For
FAST FOOD

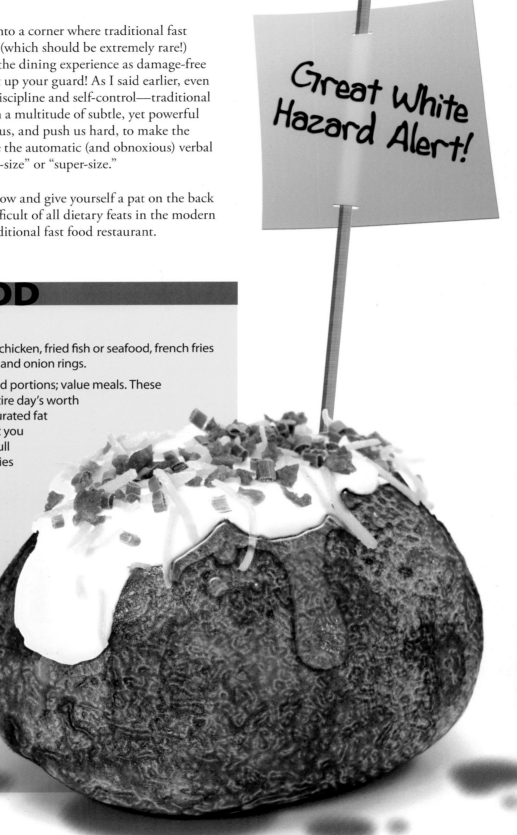

Strictly Avoid:

➤ Fried foods in any form—fried chicken, fried fish or seafood, french fries or other fried potato products, and onion rings.

➤ Oversized, biggie or super-sized portions; value meals. These options frequently have an entire day's worth of calories, not to mention saturated fat and sodium. Keep in mind that you would typically have to run a full marathon to burn off the calories in just one of those meals!

➤ Biscuits, croissants.

➤ All sugary beverages.

➤ Anything with cheese or bacon on it, especially in combination. Those ingredients can get you hooked!

➤ Any desserts other than fresh fruit.

➤ Milkshakes, dessert coffee beverages, smoothies.

➤ Loaded baked potatoes.

➤ Bread sticks.

Great White Hazard Alert!

Specific Rules For Fast Food Restaurants

The healthier options can vary depending on the "type" of fast food chain. Follow these guidelines depending on where you unavoidably end up.

Specific Rules For

BURGER CHAINS

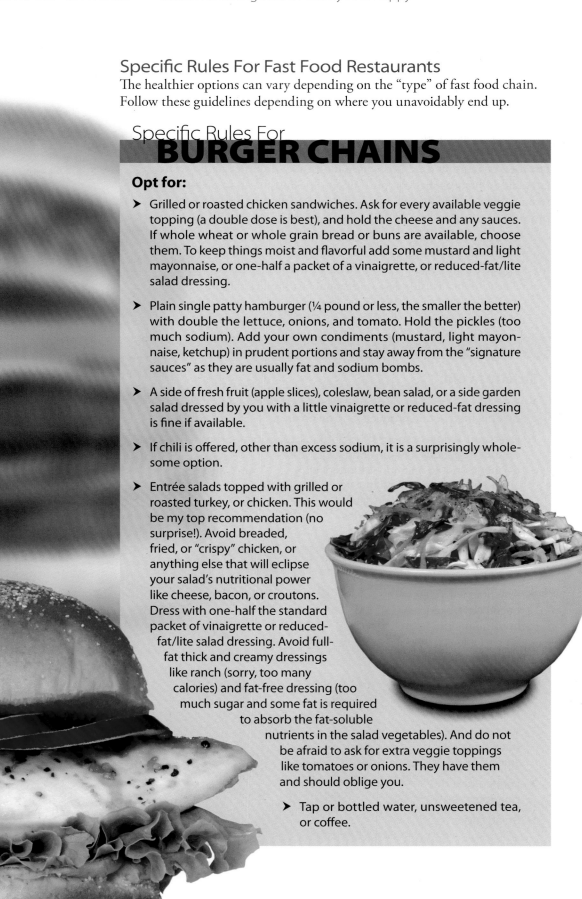

Opt for:

➤ Grilled or roasted chicken sandwiches. Ask for every available veggie topping (a double dose is best), and hold the cheese and any sauces. If whole wheat or whole grain bread or buns are available, choose them. To keep things moist and flavorful add some mustard and light mayonnaise, or one-half a packet of a vinaigrette, or reduced-fat/lite salad dressing.

➤ Plain single patty hamburger (¼ pound or less, the smaller the better) with double the lettuce, onions, and tomato. Hold the pickles (too much sodium). Add your own condiments (mustard, light mayonnaise, ketchup) in prudent portions and stay away from the "signature sauces" as they are usually fat and sodium bombs.

➤ A side of fresh fruit (apple slices), coleslaw, bean salad, or a side garden salad dressed by you with a little vinaigrette or reduced-fat dressing is fine if available.

➤ If chili is offered, other than excess sodium, it is a surprisingly wholesome option.

➤ Entrée salads topped with grilled or roasted turkey, or chicken. This would be my top recommendation (no surprise!). Avoid breaded, fried, or "crispy" chicken, or anything else that will eclipse your salad's nutritional power like cheese, bacon, or croutons. Dress with one-half the standard packet of vinaigrette or reduced-fat/lite salad dressing. Avoid full-fat thick and creamy dressings like ranch (sorry, too many calories) and fat-free dressing (too much sugar and some fat is required to absorb the fat-soluble nutrients in the salad vegetables). And do not be afraid to ask for extra veggie toppings like tomatoes or onions. They have them and should oblige you.

➤ Tap or bottled water, unsweetened tea, or coffee.

Specific Rules For
CHICKEN CHAINS

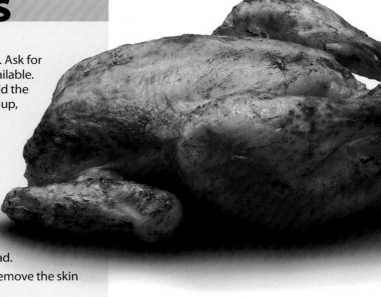

Opt for:

➤ Grilled or roasted chicken breast sandwiches or wraps. Ask for whole wheat or whole grain bread, buns, or wraps if available. Top with as many and as much veggies as possible. Hold the cheese. Season with mustard, light mayonnaise, ketchup, BBQ sauce, or reduced-fat dressing.

➤ Grilled chicken breast.

➤ BBQ chicken sandwich.

➤ Chicken salad sandwich if made with light or non-fat mayonnaise.

➤ Entrée salads if offered. (See *Specific Rules For Burger Chains* for more information.)

➤ Any of the following sides: green beans, corn on the cob, coleslaw, sweet kernel corn, collard greens, side salad.

➤ If breaded fried chicken is the only possibility for you, remove the skin before you eat it (this cuts the fat calories in half).

➤ Tap or bottled water, unsweetened tea, or coffee.

Specific Rules For
TACO CHAINS

Opt for:

➤ Grilled chicken soft taco.

➤ Bean burrito.

➤ Grilled chicken burrito.

➤ Fresco-style bean or chicken burrito or soft taco.

➤ Choose salsa, guacamole, green tomatillo sauces, or reduced-fat sour cream for condiments.

➤ Tap or bottled water, unsweetened tea, or coffee.

Specific Rules For
PIZZA CHAINS

Opt for:

➤ Thin crust or whole wheat/whole grain crust (the latter now available in some chains).

➤ Veggie toppings (the more the better), or grilled chicken with veggies.

➤ One slice of large or two slices of medium is suitable for portions.

➤ If reduced-calorie options are available (like Pizza Hut's Fit 'n Delicious line), they are also a good choice. Stick to chicken and veggie toppings, however.

Sit-Down Restaurants

Now let's master the next major sector of the restaurant food world—casual, sit-down dining. This popular form of dining is just behind fast food as the most common manner of eating outside of the home. We will confront many of the same challenges we faced in our fast food adventures, but because we are already warmed up and will be applying strategies that are familiar to you, this section promises to be smooth sailing.

My gut tells me that this is a good time to take a quick look at our road map and review the cardinal rules for healthy eating. Better yet, let's focus on the foods we are trying to bring to the table—the right foods—and then those we are trying to keep off the table—the wrong foods.

The Right Foods Include:

➤ Healthy fats—Monounsaturated fats from extra virgin olive oil, canola oil, nuts, seeds and avocados; omega 3 fats from seafood, especially oily fish like salmon and whole soy foods.

➤ A variety of fruits and vegetables (not white potatoes though!).

➤ Wholesome, fiber-rich (lower glycemic) starches—physically intact whole grains like brown rice, barley and quinoa, beans, sweet potatoes, winter squash and whole grain breads.

➤ Healthy proteins—fish, shellfish, turkey, chicken, beans, whole soy foods and eggs.

The Wrong Foods Include:

➤ The Great White Hazards—white flour products like breads, rolls, biscuits and pizza crust, white rice, white potatoes and sweets.

➤ Foods high in saturated fats—red meat (especially fatty cuts and processed varieties like bacon and sausage), whole dairy products like cheese, cream and butter, and palm oil.

➤ Foods that contain trans fats or oxidized fats—stick margarine, shortening and deep fried foods.

➤ Sugary beverages—soda, fruit drinks, sweet tea and dessert beverages.

> *"One of the distinct advantages of sit-down restaurants is that you generally have a more direct say-so in how your food is prepared and what specifically goes onto your plate."*

Take Charge Of Your Plate

One of the distinct advantages of sit-down restaurants is that you generally have a more direct say-so in how your food is prepared and what specifically goes onto your plate. This brings me to the most important over-arching piece of advice I can offer to help you eat healthfully in this context: Be proactive in your selections and fully prepared to call the shots. Like I have said repeatedly—YOU need to be the person in control of your nutritional environment. YOU need to be the person who dictates exactly what foods you will consume. Because if you don't, you will likely fail–and it is as simple as that. So put your feet down firmly, hold your head up high, and get ready to take charge of your plate!

Beware Of The Obstacles At Sit-Down Restaurants

As the commander-in-chief of your diet, you need to be reminded of the obstacles you will frequently run into that can cause you to stumble and fall, sabotaging your health and your good intentions:

➤ Big/Oversized Portions. Beware that portions in casual dining chains are even bigger and more risky than those served in fast food chains. Based on standard serving sizes as published by the USDA, most entrées (and even many appetizers), provide two to four servings. Portion pressure will be your biggest threat.

➤ High Glycemic Carbs. White bread, white potatoes, white pasta and white rice are the staple starches across all casual dining restaurants. Yes, the Great White Hazards are far and wide.

➤ High Caloric Density. Fried foods, fatty meats like hamburger, ribs and bacon, cream sauces, and cheese and more cheese are everywhere.

➤ Excess Sodium. Most restaurant foods are high in sodium, especially sauces, cheese, Chinese foods and dishes that come with processed meat (bacon, ham, sausage, etc.).

➤ Ultra Palatable Foods. Of course, the usual suspects like chili cheese fries, onion rings smothered in ranch, bacon cheeseburgers, loaded nachos and potato skins, creamy pasta dishes and oversized, decadent desserts will be omnipresent.

➤ Variety In Foods And Flavor. Oh so many choices with a bonanza of flavors!

➤ Low In Fiber (Highly Processed). This is actually one of the bright spots. Typically you will find a nice selection of fiber-rich vegetables and even some bean-based dishes. Unfortunately, whole grains are still far out-numbered by refined grains like white bread and white rice (which drives me nuts!).

➤ Excessive Saturated Fats. Burgers, fatty steaks, ribs, cheesy appetizers and entrees, deep-fried foods and dishes amped up with bacon and sausage are core offerings for casual dining chains.

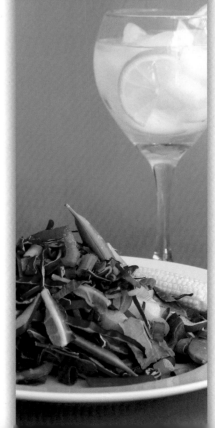

Create The "PERFECT PLATE"

I am a big believer in simple visuals for staying on track with healthy eating and was thrilled when the USDA adopted the "My Plate" icon to replace the confusing and essentially useless "food pyramid." When I sit down to order a meal, I always aspire to create the "perfect plate"—with one-half of the plate filled with vegetables, one quarter filled with lean protein, and one quarter with a healthy starch (whole grains, beans, sweet potatoes, etc). If I can't find a healthy starch, I substitute more vegetables. If I am feeling particularly veggie, I will get the entire plate covered in vegetables and top them with some lean protein (as in an entrée salad).

General Rules For Sit-Down Restaurants

Now let's sit down, put this all together, and build a meal that is good for you in your favorite casual dining outlet. For success, follow these dining out "best practices."

Number 1: Exercise Your...

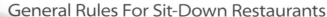

PORTION CONTROL

As I already exclaimed, this will be your biggest challenge. Fortunately, there are several simple strategies you can deploy to fight and defeat the portion monster you will undoubtedly face. It starts by personally acknowledging that you are going to be served more than you need. Just because you see others cleaning their plates does not mean it is normal or appropriate.

➤ To stay on target with portions when you order, use your very own hands. Limit what you plan to eat (and ideally order) to what would fit in your two hands cupped together minus any fruit and veggies (no need to limit fruits or veggies).

➤ Request that your server package half of your meal in a take-home box before you are served. This way you get two meals for the price of one! As an alternative, request they serve you a smaller portion than normal. I do this often when traveling because doggie bags in hotels and planes are a nuisance. The servers look at me like I'm crazy, which I especially enjoy because it is affirmation that I am in control. (As I'm sure you've suspected, when it comes to my nutritional environment, I am a control freak.)

➤ Consider an appetizer as your main dish. Be careful though! If you are in a casual dining chain like Applebee's, Ruby Tuesday, TGIFridays, Chili's, etc., where oversized and ultra palatable things like buffalo wings, fried mozzarella sticks, or loaded nacho and potato skins are the options, this would not be a wise choice.

➤ Share an entrée with your dining partner.

➤ Do your best to avoid buffet offerings and all-you-can-eat restaurants. Studies confirm the more quantity and variety available to us; the more we eat.

➤ Look for "petite," "mini," "small" or "half-portion" entrée selections. Thankfully, these more sanely-sized options are becoming more common.

➤ Refrain from ordering menu items with big fat descriptions like "giant," "grande," "jumbo," or "supreme."

➤ Wear more tightly fitting clothes. If you do, chances are you will get a "gut feeling" when you have had enough.

➤ Although this can be very tough, don't clean your plate. If you eat half of the food served to you, you will be eating the same amount as restaurant patrons did 30 years ago (and they were a lot leaner than we are now).

Number 2: Stop Consuming The...
GREAT WHITE HAZARDS

➤ Request that the basket of bread (unless it is whole grain) or chips not be brought to your table, or have them removed as soon as you sit down. I always do this because I know it is otherwise impossible not to partake.

➤ If white potatoes, white rice, or white pasta are the default side for your entrée, ask to substitute a vegetable, some beans, or a side salad. Also inquire about the availability of brown rice.

➤ Avoid pasta entrees. Most have three full servings, which is a huge load of white flour!

➤ Always order whole grain bread instead of white bread when available.

➤ If biscuits, rolls, croissant, or bread sticks come with your order, ask that they be held. Remember if it's not there, it's not an option!

Number 3: Plan Ahead And...
REIN IN YOUR APPETITE

The hungrier we are, the more we tend to order, serve ourselves, and ultimately eat. Take heed—do not arrive at a restaurant famished. It is especially high risk to refrain from eating your meals earlier in the day to "save up" for your eating-out meal. Take advantage of these simple strategies to quiet a ravenous appetite before your meal arrives.

➤ Eat a light and healthy snack an hour before you expect to dine. Something with some fiber, protein, and a bit of fat would be the smartest choice. A few apple slices spread with a little peanut butter or a piece of fruit with a small handful of nuts is ideal.

➤ Order a side salad, or a cup or bowl of a broth or tomato-based soup as a starter. Studies confirm you will eat less of your entrée if you do.

➤ Drink a large glass of water before your meal arrives. This quick and easy tactic has also been shown in clinical studies to help you eat less.

➤ Pay close attention to your "stomach" and how hungry you really are. Studies repeatedly show we are lousy judges of "true hunger" and more often eat based on external environmental cues versus authentic hunger. Real hunger manifests as a deep pit in the stomach, not a sensation in the throat, mouth, or head.

Number 4: Load Up On…
FRUITS & VEGGIES

Fruits and vegetables are the nutritional megastars and one of the most powerful weapons available for fighting fat. Earlier in the book, I discussed the unique power of big volume foods to shut off hunger, and fruits and vegetables, because of their hefty load of fiber and water, are the "volumizing" superstars. If you want to "eat more, but weigh less"—strive to fill half of your plate with these almighty and unrivaled slimming gifts straight from Mother Nature.

➤ Carefully review the entire menu to see the full variety of vegetables offered. This includes vegetable sides that come with entrees that do not interest you and a la carte offerings (always the very first thing I do when handed a menu). Do not be afraid to ask for vegetable substitutions or additions! I do it all the time.

➤ Select an appetizer that features fruit and/or vegetables (no white potatoes!). Side or small salads with dressing on the side or vegetable-based soups are also a fantastic choice (not creamy or cheesy ones of course).

➤ Choose an entrée salad as your main dish, as I often do. Do not hesitate to ask for extra veggies—like double the carrots, peppers, or tomatoes. Hold any croutons, cheese, or bacon bits, and get the dressing on the side.

➤ Substitute vegetable sides for white potatoes, white rice, and pasta sides.

➤ Order extra vegetable sides or a double order of the vegetable that comes with your dish.

➤ If available, consider fresh fruit or fruit salad for your dessert.

➤ Select sweet potatoes over white potatoes—sweet potato fries are a better choice (and more delicious) than regular fries.

➤ Remember that white potatoes and corn do not count as vegetables in my book. We consume entirely too much of them, especially as french fries and processed corn products, and not nearly enough of the other "non-starchy" vegetables.

Number 5: Always Remember To…
DO YOUR FATS RIGHT

Remember that fat need not be a bad thing. Have your fat and eat it too, but be sure you choose the right type of fat. It is the type of fat that you eat that really matters, especially for your heart and arteries. Your goals are to bring the good fats (monounsaturated and omega 3 fats) onto your plate and keep the bad fats (saturated and trans fats) off of your plate.

➤ Request that your food be prepared in olive oil or canola oil.

➤ If you are having bread (hopefully whole grain only) with your meal, ask for a little olive oil to dip it in versus using butter or margarine.

➤ Request that cream, butter and cheese-based sauces, salad dressings, and gravy be served on the side so you can control the portions. This is especially important if you are having an entrée salad, which will typically have hundreds of calories (up to 600+) from the salad dressing—talk about raining on a healthy parade!

➤ Request an olive oil or canola oil-based vinaigrette for your salads. Reduced-fat or light dressings are acceptable choices, but not the full-fat thick ones like ranch, blue cheese, or thousand island.

➤ Strictly avoid fried foods in any form. Avoid selections that list "fried," "breaded," "crispy," or "crunchy" in their descriptions. If you are not sure if a food is fried or not, ask before you order it.

➤ Avoid selections that come with cream-based or cheese-based sauces, or at least get them on the side.

➤ Avoid cheese all together, especially options "smothered" in cheese. These choices virtually guarantee too many calories, saturated fats, and sodium.

➤ Do not order anything with "alfredo" in its description. This is a dirty word.

➤ Avoid fatty cuts of meat—burgers, fatty steaks (T-bones, rib eyes, porterhouse, New York strip, Prime rib), meat loaf, bacon, ribs, and sausage. If you must have meat, choose a prudent portion—six ounces of a lean cut (filet, tenderloin, or sirloin).

➤ Look for options providing omega 3 fats—seafood, especially oily fish like salmon, tuna and trout, or whole soy foods like tofu, tempeh, or edamame are fantastic.

➤ Opt for entrees that are grilled, broiled, baked, roasted, or pan-seared.

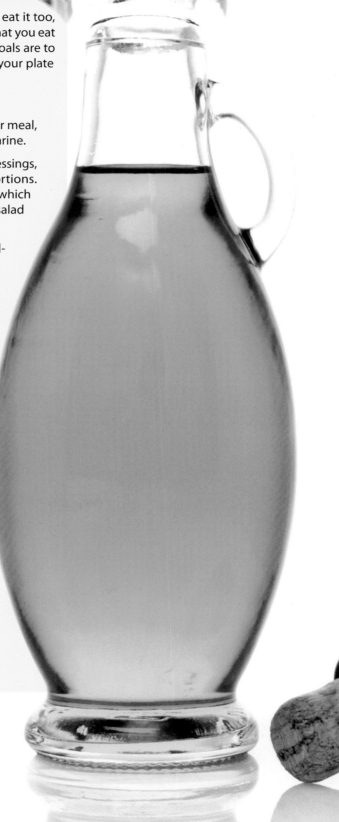

Number 6: Choose A Healthy, Lower...
GLYCEMIC STARCH

Unlike the Great White Hazards, these carbs are good to your heart and your mid-section.

➤ Look carefully for physically intact grains like brown rice, wild rice, barley, quinoa, or farro. They are becoming increasingly available in restaurants.

➤ Select sweet potatoes over white potatoes.

➤ If whole wheat or multigrain pasta is available, it is a better choice than white pasta.

➤ Winter squashes like butternut or spaghetti squash are highly nutritious starchy sides if available. Cauliflower "mock mashed potatoes" are delicious if offered.

➤ Beans in any form (except refried beans) are awesome. Go for bean soups, bean salads, bean cakes, or any other bean sides.

Number 7: Select A...
HEALTHY PROTEIN

➤ Seafood including fish or shellfish are excellent choices because they provide healthy omega 3 fats and negligible saturated fats. Americans are not consuming optimal amounts of seafood, so this would be my top recommendation for a healthy protein. Of course do not even consider ruining such a healthy thing by getting it breaded or fried. Order it grilled, broiled, baked, blackened, pan-seared, poached, or steamed. Seafood is always my top protein choice.

➤ Lean poultry like chicken or turkey is also a fine option. Try it roasted, baked, or grilled and if it comes with the skin on, remove it before you eat it. Steer clear of breaded or fried poultry options.

➤ Vegetarian selections like bean dishes, tofu, or tempeh are great for you and the environment.

➤ If you just have to have some red meat (which includes pork, too), be sure to select the leanest cuts (tenderloin, filet, or sirloin) and be mindful that a "normal serving" of cooked red meat is just four ounces or the size of a deck of cards.

Have It Your Way Or No Way: Specific Rules For Sit-Down Restaurants

As I did with fast foods, here are my more focused recommendations for the most popular types of casual dining restaurants.

Dr. Ann's Specific Rules For…
MEXICAN

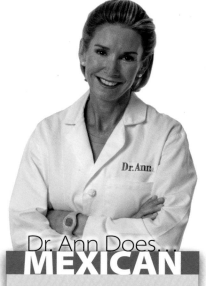

The foods that play a starring role in traditional Mexican cuisine fit beautifully in the repertoire for healthy dining, including: lots of tomatoes, beans, corn tortillas, a variety of peppers, onions, avocado, and a rich array of flavorful herbs and spices. Unfortunately, "Americanized" Mexican food all too often gets transformed into fatty, calorie-rich fare that is turbo-charged with sodium thanks to loads of greasy meats, cheese, sour cream, and salt. All of this is made even worse with lots of frying. If Mexican is on your mind for lunch or dinner, say hola! to these tips:

➤ Just say no to the complementary basket of oily tortilla chips (and the endless refills). Tell the server not to bring them to the table. Get a side salad instead or a cup of tortilla soup sans the tortillas.

➤ Avoid all the fried stuff–hard tacos, chimichangas, chile rellenos, and those ridiculously extravagant and edible taco salad bowls.

➤ Customize, customize, customize—build your meal a la carte. Typical Mexican "platters" are overwhelming in calories with some serving up more than you need for the entire day! A la carte is the only way I do Mexican unless the menu features "healthy" options.

➤ Opt for chicken, vegetable, bean, or seafood entrees over meat and cheese options.

➤ Look for plain beans versus refried beans, brown rice versus white rice, and corn tortillas or whole wheat tortillas versus white flour ones.

➤ Build your own burrito or soft tacos (two is enough) with healthy stuffings, including: grilled chicken, fish or shrimp, any and every possible vegetable, no cheese or a little bit, and plain beans. Season with the right condiments, below.

➤ The right condiments are salsa (awesome, so pile it on!), pico de gallo, guacamole (yummy, healthy fat), diced hot peppers and tomatillo sauce. Skip the sour cream and cheese sauces.

Even if your burrito is whole wheat (and absolutely if it is white flour)–tear away the excess tortilla in the "folded" section of the wrap and throw it away. You will never miss this totally redundant flour, and it gets soggy anyway.

Dr. Ann Does…
MEXICAN

On The Border is the most common casual dining Mexican chain. Here is what I would order to do my Mexican right.

The Pico Shrimp Tacos (comes with two) with extra pico de gallo, a double order of grilled vegetables, and a side of black beans. I would also request a spoonful of guacamole (I love fresh-made guacamole!) to mix with my beans and veggies.

Or…

The Jalapeño Barbecue Salmon with a double order of grilled vegetables and a side of black beans. I would request a mound of pico de gallo on the side with a spoonful of guacamole.

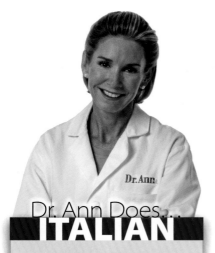

Dr. Ann Does…
ITALIAN

Olive Garden is by far the most common Italian restaurant chain. If I were ordering from their menu, it would be:

➤ A side garden salad as my appetizer with extra carrots and tomatoes, and dressing on the side (no croutons); or a bowl of minestrone soup (only if I was really hungry, and I would not eat most of the pasta in it).

➤ Herb-grilled salmon or Venetian apricot chicken. Both come with a generous portion of non-starchy vegetables and no pasta.

Dr. Ann's Specific Rules For…
ITALIAN

Just like its Mexican compatriot, the original bones of this lovable gastronomy were worthy of many nutritional accolades. Unfortunately, our modern, westernized ways tend to crowd out the good stuff and tempt us with way too much of the bad. Oversized portions of white flour pasta drenched with cheesy and creamy sauces, and white bread out the wazoo tend to rule. Thankfully, however, you can go Italian and go healthy too.

➤ If you are particularly hungry, order a side salad or a bowl of minestrone soup quick, and forget any bread, especially garlic bread (white flour and butter bombs). Command the server to keep the bread basket and any bread sides off of your table and plate—you'll want to thank him later.

➤ If you're really drooling over the pasta options, order a half portion or have them box up half before it arrives. If whole wheat or multigrain options are available, (highly unlikely though) choose them.

➤ Opt for tomato-based pasta sauces like marinara (loaded with lycopene) or red clam sauce versus the cream or cheese-based (really fattening) ones. This means be afraid of anything "alfredo." Pesto is fine in small amounts.

➤ Totally veg out with any vegetables—fresh salads, antipasto, broccoli, asparagus, mushrooms, bell peppers, and diced tomatoes are Mediterranean favorites and almost always on the menu. Be bold and ask for extra veggies and veggie substitutions, especially in lieu of pasta sides.

➤ Grilled shrimp, fish, or chicken without sauce or on the side are far superior choices than breaded and fried versions. Stay away from beef, pork, and "filled pasta" entrees.

➤ If you want pizza (which I honestly do not recommend—too much flour), refer to page 63 for guidance.

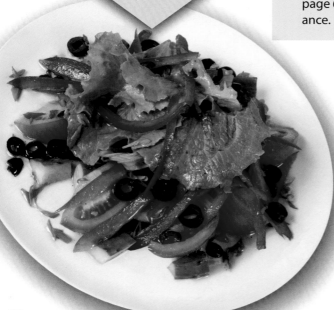

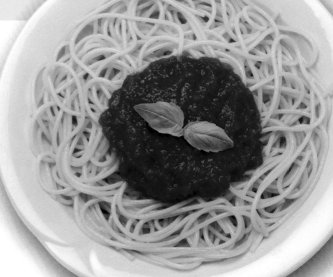

Dr. Ann's Specific Rules For…
CHINESE & ASIAN

Traditional Asian cuisine is steeped in nutritional excellence and likely why most people automatically perceive this ethnic favorite, even the sweet and sour pork, to be healthy. Regrettably, American-Asian is not Asian-Asian. Platters piled high with breaded and deep-fried pork, chicken, or beef, the occasional vegetable, and a mountain of fried rice are literally worlds away from steamed fish or tofu served with a little steamed rice and a big bouquet of Asian vegetables. Relative to the other Americanized ethnic foods however, Asian fare generally does have less bad fat, but you pay for it with more sodium. If Asian feeds your dining fancies, don't freak—simply follow these guidelines and speak up when you order, and you will come out just fine, even from the neighborhood take-out joint.

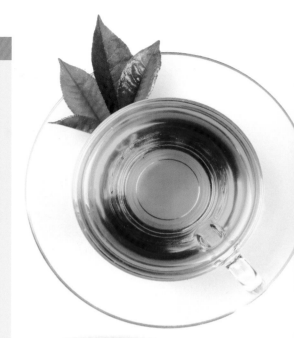

➤ Choose entrees that feature steamed or stir-fried vegetables and/or unbreaded chicken or seafood. Avoid any deep-fried or breaded selections and those that come with pasta or noodles (unless the noodles are made from brown rice or buckwheat like soba noodles). No chow mein (fried noodle) dishes. If you are not sure if your entrée is fried or breaded, inquire!

➤ Opt for steamed versus fried rice and of course brown rice if available.

➤ Request "heavy" on the vegetables and "light" on the chicken or seafood in your selections.

➤ Hold any crispy noodles or fried wontons that come as garnish or toppings.

➤ Give the tofu (not deep-fried) a go for your protein source. You will be amazed how delicious it can be.

➤ Stick with unfried summer or spring rolls versus traditional fried egg rolls.

➤ If red meat is a must, beef with broccoli or beef with stir-fry vegetables is your best bet. (No "crispy" beef.)

➤ Choose low sodium soy sauce or a small portion of duck or hoisin sauce to boost flavors. Rice vinegar and wasabi are fine, too.

➤ Make a toast to your dining partner with some unsweetened green tea.

Dr. Ann's Specific Rules For American…

GRILLS & DINERS

Over the past three decades, "dinner houses" like TGIFridays, Ruby Tuesday, Applebee's, and Chili's have emerged as one of the most popular places to gather with friends and family to indulge in classic American food. With warm and inviting atmospheres and menus with something to suit everyone's palate, people have flocked to them. Their enormous array of options is equally matched, however, with appalling amounts of calories and grease. Because of the preponderance of fried foods, fatty steaks and ribs, cheese-cheese-cheese, and rich creamy sauces, it is especially challenging to keep the calories in your meal to an appropriate level. Thankfully, with a little awareness, an eye towards healthy selections (always available), the gumption to request healthy substitutions, and staunch adherence to portion control—I promise you can have your meal and eat it, too!

➤ Be exceedingly wary with your appetizer selections. Dinner houses are infamous for calorie and fat-laden starters like loaded potato skins, onion rings with ranch, fried cheese, and Buffalo wings that make damage control almost impossible. These "classic American" appetizers encompass the "classic" features that will hijack appetite control and promote food addiction—lots of fat with lots of salt. Your entrée will be coming with plenty of food and calories so if you must—make your starter a side salad or a cup of a non-creamy soup. If you do give in, know that you will likely be getting 600–1,000 plus calories before your main dish and that you will have to run six to ten miles just to burn off your starter.

Dr. Ann's Specific Rules For American…
GRILLS & DINERS (CONT'D)

➤ Along with a broad selection of vegetable sides, (yoohoo!) another healthy highlight on the menu will be entrée salads. Select those that offer the most vegetables and top your salad with some lean protein like grilled chicken, shrimp, or salmon. Stay away from salads that come with anything crispy or fried or request a substitution. Hold the bacon, croutons, fried noodles, and tortilla strips, and go light on the cheese. Always (certainly you know this by now) request that your dressing be on the side, and be careful with the one you select. Vinaigrettes or reduced-fat options are best. I know from lots of experience that half or less of the dressing served on the side will be plenty if you toss the salad thoroughly.

➤ Look for entrees featuring clean and lean protein like grilled or pan-seared, unbreaded chicken breast, fish, or sirloin steak. Grilled salmon (go omega 3!) is almost always available.

➤ Select as many non-starchy vegetables like broccoli, asparagus, zucchini, and green beans, or a veggie medley for your sides in lieu of potatoes in any form, or pasta. Again, this is a true bright spot in most American dinner houses. If brown rice or beans are available go for them.

➤ A bowl of chili (sans cheese) is a wholesome choice, and you can make it even better by pairing it with a garden salad.

➤ Stay away from sandwiches, burgers, (most have 900 plus calories) fatty steaks, ribs, pasta dishes, and entrees that come with cheese. If you feel tempted, request to view the nutritional info for the selections so you at least know the calorie fix you will be getting yourself into.

➤ Opt for half, light, or petite portions, which are now frequently available—hurray!

➤ To make things really quick and easy—go straight to the menu items featured as "healthy" or "smart" choices and forget even looking at the remainder of the menu. How simple is that!

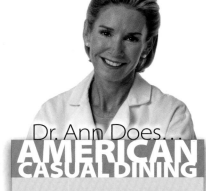

Dr. Ann Does…
AMERICAN CASUAL DINING

Here is what my order would look like in the three most common dinner house chains.

Ruby Tuesday
Lunch: A big entrée salad from the Garden bar as per page 62. (See *Specific Rules For Burger Chains* for more information.)

Dinner: Grilled salmon with side of steamed broccoli, roasted spaghetti squash (healthy starch), and grilled asparagus or grilled zucchini.

Applebee's
Lunch: Try black bean soup with half portion grilled oriental chicken salad with dressing on the side.

Dinner: Garlic-herb salmon with house salad and side of seasonal veggies, or grilled shrimp n' spinach salad with dressing on the side.

Chili's
Lunch: Caribbean salad with grilled chicken and dressing on the side.

Dinner: Lighter choice grilled salmon with steamed broccoli and substitution of black beans for the rice.

Enjoy Your **JAVA**

With the exception of those who are pregnant or intolerant of the stimulating properties of caffeine, coffee is not only a remarkably safe (and delicious!) beverage, mounting science is discovering that it conveys significant health benefits too. A report in the *American Journal of Epidemiology* that followed over 38,000 adults for a 13 year period found that those who drank one or more cups of coffee a day were 50% less likely to get cancer of the mouth or throat compared to non-coffee drinkers.

And in another report we had promising news that our brains may benefit too. In this study, researchers reported that people who drank three to five cups of coffee a day were 65% less likely to develop Alzheimer's disease than those who drank little to none. Bear in mind we already have strong evidence that regular coffee consumption decreases the risk of Parkinson's disease, type 2 diabetes, liver cancer, and gallstones, while enhancing mental performance, mood, and physical endurance. For those of you like me who love to wake up to a good cup of coffee this is joyful java news.

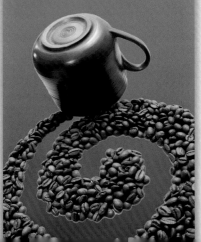

Rethink Your Drink

It is now widely accepted that sugary beverages are the most fattening of all forms of calories and have subsequently played a leading role in the obesity epidemic. In fact, of all the things you could do to lose weight, dumping sugary beverages appears to provide the single greatest return for your efforts! The unique propensity of sweet liquids like soda, fruit drinks, and dessert coffees to tip the scale in the wrong direction is due to at least four separate and distinct, particularly fattening features. This quadruple threat to your waistline occurs through the following means:

1. Liquid calories do not suppress the human appetite like solid food calories. Despite the fact that they can be loaded with calories, we do not seem to be less hungry or to eat less after consuming them. Somehow liquid calories pass under the radar of the body's satiety (full feeling) mechanisms, and do not elicit the hunger-quieting signals that real foods do.

2. Sugary beverages launch blood sugar (glucose) levels up high and fast, followed by a steep and sudden drop that can trigger hunger.

3. Sugary beverages also quickly drive up blood fructose levels, which incite a number of adverse consequences that can promote weight gain. This is emerging as the primary culprit in the adverse health effects observed with regular consumption of sugary beverages.

4. Sipping relative to chewing provides minimal "orosensory satiety" and makes it considerably easier to take in excess calories quickly and effortlessly.

The result? A perfect storm of distinctly obesogenic calories that go down fast!

Keep in mind that standard beverage servings in sit down, casual dining chains are typically 14-22 ounces. If you ask for a sugary selection, like soda, you will be getting 175-275 calories and 11-17 teaspoons of sugar even before your free refill. Those drinks on the house are a menace!

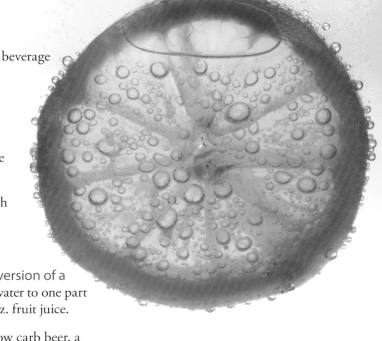

To stay on track and avoid a bellyful of calories, select a beverage that will fill you up, but not fill you out.

➤ Water

➤ Unsweetened hot or cold tea

➤ Unsweetened coffee (I recommend that everyone avoid caffeine after 2:00 PM).

➤ Sparkling water/seltzer (This is very refreshing with a twist of lemon or lime).

➤ Skim or reduced-fat milk

➤ If plain water is just too plain for you, order my version of a "healthy soft drink"—three parts seltzer/sparking water to one part 100% fruit juice. In other words, 9 oz. seltzer to 3 oz. fruit juice.

➤ If you desire an alcoholic beverage—a light or low carb beer, a glass of wine, or liquor with a non-caloric mixer is the best choice.

As an additional, positive incentive, recognize that reducing the intake of liquid calories does not seem to make us hungrier, as is the case with reducing the intake of solid-food calories.

What About Dessert?

If eating out is something you do regularly—forget dessert and make it a habit. You know by now you'll have enough calorie challenges in your main dish alone, and other than fresh fruit or dark chocolate, there is no way sweet restaurant treats can be healthy. If you are dining out for a special circumstance like a birthday or an anniversary, an occasional sweet splurge is fine.

Because the first bite always tastes the very best, with each subsequent spoonful providing less palatal pleasure (thanks to sensory-specific satiety), try sharing a dessert with your dining partner or partners, so you can get your sweet fix for less calories (and less money). For additional motivation, keep in mind that many casual dining restaurant chains offer desserts that pack a whopping 800 to 1,000+ calories that come along with one to two days worth of artery-jolting saturated fat. Chocolate cakes, cheesecakes, brownie and blondie features, sundaes, and chocolate chip pies are particularly nefarious choices due to their over-the-top caloric and fatty exuberance.

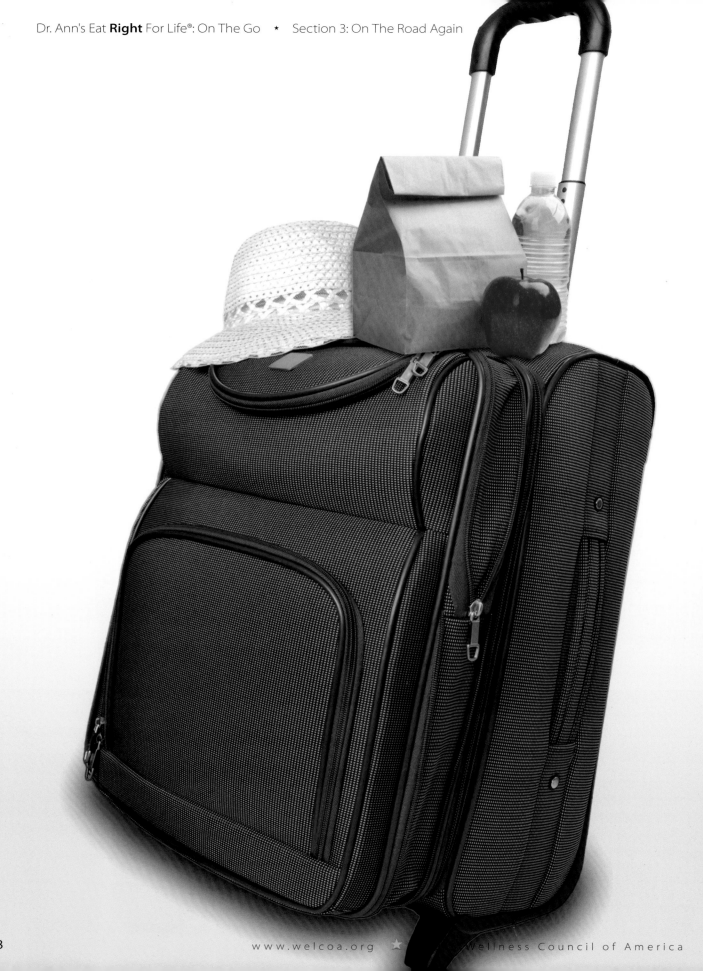

On The Road Again

On The Road Again

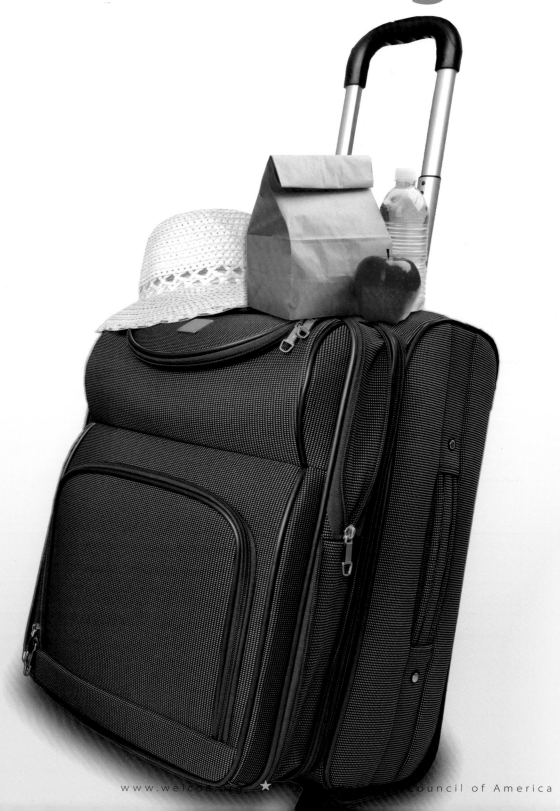

For those of you like me who find yourself regularly on the road and in the air, it gives me great pleasure to steer you away from the obstacles and down the smooth pathway to healthy eating while traveling. In addition to the toxic food culture you will invariably face, traveling comes with additional roadblocks including time constraints and stress. With awareness, a little pre-planning, and some know-how in what constitutes healthy choices and where to find them, I promise you can arrive safely and nutritionally sound.

Up In The Air

Let's begin with air travel and eating on the airplane. Food and beverage selections offered on planes are highly consistent across all major airlines so this will be very straightforward.

➤ The complimentary snack will be pretzels, peanuts, or shortbread cookies. Forget the pretzels (white flour turbo-charged with sodium) and cookies (white flour, sugar, salt, bad fat) and opt for the peanuts, which are by far the nutritionally superior selection (seven different great-for-your heart nutrients). And for goodness' sake—if you are not hungry, say no to them or stash them for later when real hunger hits.

➤ Of course, you can also pack your own healthy snacks. Quick and easy, air-friendly options include: nuts, wasabi peas, or soy nuts in a ziplock bag; a piece of fresh fruit wrapped, courtesy of nature, in its own skin; (unpeeled apples, bananas, oranges, etc.) individually wrapped dark chocolate squares; string cheese, granola bars (I prefer Kashi brand); or fresh cut veggies in a ziplock bag with a healthy dip, such as a small container of hummus.

➤ Of the complimentary beverages offered, choose water, seltzer water, or unsweetened tea or coffee. If you are lean and active, 4-6 oz. of 100% fruit juice (this excludes cranberry cocktail) is acceptable. Seltzer water spiked with a little 100% fruit juice is also fine. If the tomato juice or bloody mary mix were low in sodium, they would be fine, but I have yet to encounter this healthier option. Keep in mind that excess sodium and air travel are a horrible combination for bloating and fluid retention.

➤ Please remember that the more water you drink during air travel, the better you will look and feel. Airplanes are notoriously dry and the extra water keeps the mucous membranes of your nose and mouth from drying out. Dry mucus membranes make it easier for germs to get into your system and leave you feeling miserable. The extra hydration will also help mitigate the dreaded travel bloat. I always carry my BPA-free plastic water bottle with me and fill it with tap water once I get through airport security.

If lunch is in the air, my first choice is dinner leftovers. Provided it will be less than two hours from fridge to my mouth, if I have leftovers—it is a done deal!

➤ If your departure flight (leaving home) overlaps with breakfast or lunchtime, do a little pre-planning and pack your own meal. All airlines now charge for meals on domestic flights and unfortunately the taste and nutritional quality are awful. Brown bagging in the air is standard flight procedure for me. I know I can make a meal far healthier and tastier than those pre-fab, processed, boxed things. My preferred breakfast-on-the-fly is plain yogurt and berries. I simply dump some Greek-style plain yogurt into a plastic container, top it with some frozen berries, and if I have some in stock, garnish it with my homemade granola. I carefully seal down the top (and triple check it), place it in a ziplock bag for extra spill protection, and grab a plastic spoon and napkin when I get to the airport. Other simple grab-and-go breakfast options include:

- 1 ½ ounces (a healthy handful) of nuts of choice in a sealed ziplock bag with a piece of fresh fruit
- Two part-skim mozzarella cheese sticks with a piece of fresh fruit
- Two hard boiled omega 3 eggs with a piece of fresh fruit
- Two granola bars (I prefer Kashi) topped with a thin layer of peanut or almond butter and placed together like a sandwich along with a piece of fresh fruit
- One cup of finger-friendly healthy dry cereal (I like Quaker Oat Squares or Kashi Cinnamon Harvest) with a piece of fresh fruit
- 1 ½ ounces of roasted soy nuts with a piece of fresh fruit
- Two squares of dark chocolate with a banana (another favorite of mine)

➤ If lunch is in the air, my first choice is dinner leftovers. Provided it will be less than two hours from fridge to my mouth, if I have leftovers—it is a done deal. They are already packaged in a sealed to-go container, and I love leftovers! I place a small freezer pack in a ziplock bag and wrap the freezer pack and the to-go container a few times in tin foil for extra-insulation and to keep the icepack in close proximity to my food. If you have a small insulated lunch box or container that fits in your carry on, of course that works too. You may have to remove the freezer pack at the security checkpoint though.

➤ **Sandwiches are another easy and convenient in-flight lunch alternative.** Peanut butter and banana, classic PB&J, or your favorite deli meat with fresh veggies on 100% whole wheat bread are healthy choices. To keep any vegetables crisp, package them separately in a ziplock bag and add them to your sandwich when it's time to dine. Be sure to cut your sandwich in half, tightly wrap each half in plastic wrap, and place in a hard plastic sandwich container to keep it from getting smashed. To round things off nutritionally, throw in some fresh fruit or fresh cut vegetables.

➤ **Salads that work well at room temperature, such as those made with beans or hearty whole grains like brown rice or quinoa, are fantastic travel companions.** They are super-nutritious, filling, easy-to-pack in a sealed plastic container, and proudly stand alone as a balanced meal. For my favorite salad recipes that I know from experience travel nicely, go to the "free recipes" tab of my homepage (DrAnnWellness.com) and follow the links to salads. The healthy bean salad, edamame salad, rice salad primavera, and Italian quinoa salad are delicious and fit for flight. When you pull out these oh-so-healthy lunch salads, it's sure to impress your seatmates. And because healthy behaviors can be socially contagious, you can feel good about spreading the health! Don't forget to grab your plastic fork and napkin in the airport before you get on the jet way.

The Six Commandments Of
HEALTHY JET-SETTERS

Abide by these on-the-go principles for the flight to high health.

1. I will not enter the airport terminal famished, and I will always keep healthy hunger-fighting snacks in my carry-on bag for ready access.

2. Because I may be stressed, pressed for time, or bored, I will be keenly mindful of practicing self-control and prepared to totally ignore the siren calls of ice cream, donut, pastry, cookie, pretzel and candy shops. Additionally, I will strive to avoid stepping within "sniffing distance" of them.

3. If I need to eat a meal or pick one up to take on the plane, I will go straight to the nearest airport terminal map to review all of my dining options so I can make an informed, healthy decision. Better yet, I will plan to review the airport terminal map on the airport's website prior to my flight departure so I will already be familiar with the locations of the better-for-me dining spots. Keep in mind some are available as mobile apps.

4. Assuming time allows, I will happily walk briskly (no use of trains or moving walkways) to the terminal that has the dining option that best provides the tasty and healthy meal I am proactively seeking.

5. I will keep the cardinal rules of healthy eating in mind when ordering to ensure my meal will be good for me.

6. If time allows and my healthcare provider has approved, I will use my time in the airport to walk briskly as part of my goal to build in at least 30 minutes of daily physical activity even when I am on the road. I will be grateful for my carry on bags that increase the effectiveness of my airport exercise regimen. Not taking advantage of the opportunities to walk in the airport is one of my biggest pet peeves. I am always amazed at the numbers of people just sitting around—in case you don't know it, prolonged sitting is not only bad for you, but can be deadly!

> *While airport cuisine has traditionally been sorely deficient in healthy options, fresh, healthy, local, gourmet, and even organic offerings are now taking off—all thanks to consumer demand.*

Staying On Course In The Concourse

When it comes to healthy eating in the airport, I have some bad news and some great news. On the negative side, airport eating comes with a cavalcade of added stressors that can make it particularly tough to stay mindful and to execute the level of self-control healthy success demands. On top of the typical stress that naturally comes with air travel, you have to deal with carrying bags, crowds, zooming golf carts, delayed and canceled flights, and a cacophony of obtrusive noises.

At the same time, we are dealing with these distracting and unnerving pressures and stressors, we are coursing through a virtual junk food Shangri-la—bombarded on both sides by the sight and smells of an extraordinary assortment of decadent, ultra-palatable foods—Cinnabon anyone? This kind of stimulation puts even a nutritional control fanatic like me to the test. Honestly, airports are almost always where I make my nutritional blunders. I have been caught more than once "orange-handed" with Cheetos—oops!

BLUEBERRY SCONE
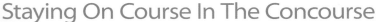

A few years back on a departure flight from a speaking engagement out west, I had an "aha!" experience with a blueberry scone that I will never forget and want to share with you. I had a very early flight departure (6:30 AM) and wanted to grab my gotta-have-it cup of coffee and some semblance of a healthy breakfast prior to boarding. Because it was so early, my only option for food was a popular coffee shop chain. As I waited in line, I quickly previewed all the possible offerings and readily realized that virtually every single one was nothing more than white flour and sugar. I had no healthy snacks with me (shame on me!) and dreaded the thought of my three and a half hour flight home on an empty, grumbling stomach. Feeling pressed for time and hungry, I made the impulse decision to go for a blueberry scone, thinking at least I would get some antioxidants from those blueberries! (Keep in mind that I never eat Great White Hazards, at least in the amounts that I was getting ready to encounter.) I ate the whole thing—all 460 calories of the white flour and sugar. About and hour and a half later, I was struck with one of the most intense hunger pains I could ever recall. Of course, I had no snacks and knew the complimentary pretzels (more white flour) would just add fuel to my burning appetite. From that point until touchdown all I could do was think about food and eating. As soon as my feet hit the terminal, I made a beeline straight to a snack bag of nuts (this time I knew better) to healthfully take the edge off of my hunger.

In retrospect, I should have known exactly what I was getting my appetite into. Scones are nothing less than biscuits on steroids with added sugar. Normally I do not make reckless food choices, but I am grateful for the experience because I definitely learned from it. In fact, now when I see those endless lines of people at coffee shop counters, many of whom I know will be ordering a Great White Hazard just like I did, all I want to do is scream out, "Don't get those appetite stimulants!"

On a much happier note, healthy change is definitely in the air and down on the ground in the airport terminals. While airport cuisine has traditionally been sorely deficient in healthy options, fresh, healthy, local, gourmet, and even organic offerings are now taking off—all thanks to consumer demand. Ten years ago, a grab-and-go whole-wheat wrap with turkey, grilled yellow bell peppers, fresh herbs and a red onion balsamic glaze was unheard of! Whether your desire is hummus and veggies on whole wheat, black bean burgers, brown rice sushi, or a made-to-order fresh cut salad—with the commitment to seek out the good while snubbing the bad, you can arrive at your final destination healthier than you left.

Beeline For Breakfast

A healthy breakfast is the perfect way to begin a busy travel day and to keep your inner cookie monster from attacking right in front of the Mrs. Fields' cookies in the next airport. To do your breakfast right, opt for:

➤ Oatmeal (now available at Starbucks). The nuts and dried fruit toppings are fine.

➤ Fresh whole fruit (apples and bananas abound) or packaged fresh fruit salad to go with an individual container of vanilla yogurt. Greek-style is best for its extra protein (I have yet to find plain yogurt available).

➤ Whole-wheat bagel (smallest size available) with some light cream cheese and berry-based spread or a whole-wheat bagel sandwich. Order your breakfast sandwich with any of the following: eggs, veggies, smoked salmon, avocados, or turkey (no cheese, bacon, sausage, or full-fat cream cheese). A whole-wheat breakfast wrap is fine too. Dunkin Donuts has an egg and veggie wrap on their "smart" menu.

➤ Whole grain cereal (Sorry, no Fruit Loops!) with 1% milk and a banana.

➤ If you prefer to dine in at a sit down restaurant—order a two-egg veggie omelet (light on the cheese) with a side of fresh fruit salad. Hold the side of toast, biscuits, or hash browns.

➤ Avoid the muffins, pastries, donuts, croissants, and scones unless you want to be sluggish and starving mid-morning.

Watch For Those MUFFINS!

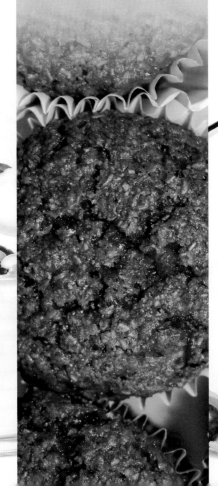

Because of the wholesome words commonly used to describe muffin offerings like "bran," "carrot-walnut," or "cranberry," these no-icing jumbo cupcakes have a healthier reputation than they deserve. Some come with upwards of 550 calories and 10 teaspoons of sugar (which makes a donut seem benign).

Do not be taken by the low-fat options either. They may contain less fat, but extra sugar is almost always added in order to compensate for the loss of flavor, making the muffins even worse for you. Fluffy refined flour in combination with sugar, no matter what its shape or name, will always be a dangerous duo.

Sensible Airport Eats For Lunch Or Dinner

Whether it is time for lunch of dinner, simply apply what you have learned in the previous parts of the book to land a good-for-you meal. My top-flight picks include:

➤ Fresh made to order salads—almost always available. Of course with lots of veggies, lean protein, dressing on the side—you know the drill.

➤ Whole grain or whole-wheat sandwiches, or wraps, with lean protein of choice and as many veggies as possible.

➤ Gourmet prepared salads made from hearty whole grains like farro, quinoa, or bulgur, or beans. Avoid pasta salads and potato salads.

➤ If you have the time and want to dine in a sit down restaurant—refer to my guidance in Section 2: *Dining Out…Happy And Healthy* (page 64).

➤ If you wind up in the food court, recognize the various outlets are definitely a mixed bag. Please keep the cardinal rules of healthy eating in mind as you survey your options. (Which means you ignore the fast food and pizza joints.) Look for a salad, Asian, or home-cooked dining establishment. Stick with a lean protein entrée (unbreaded grilled/baked chicken breast or seafood) with two or more non-starchy vegetable sides. No noodles, white rice, macaroni, or mashed potatoes.

HEALTHY SNACK STASH

Although it is best to pack your own, wholesome snacks can always be found in the terminal. Look for:

➤ Fresh fruit salads in convenient to-go plastic containers. They are now all over the airport, but I wish they were heavier on the berries!

➤ Packaged fresh raw veggies with a side of salad dressing for dipping. Dressing is usually thick and full of fat, so control it or dip into some mustard instead.

➤ Packaged nuts, any variety except the sugar-coated ones. Airport packaged nuts usually have several servings per bag, (and up to 1000 calories) so be careful!

➤ Sushi, especially brown rice sushi with vegetables and seafood.

➤ Granola bars.

➤ Beware—just like in the movie theaters, airport packaged snacks are typically jumbo-sized so be especially vigilant in keeping your hands away from the chips, cookies, and candy.

Classic Airport Pitfalls

As I have repeatedly discussed in this book, white flour, sugar and salt play a starring role in our modern day toxic food environments. Because airports represent a true microcosm of our food pop culture, you can be sure to encounter these villains wherever you go. So you can be prepared and ready to stand up to them if they strike, beware of their most popular hangouts.

Coffee Shop/Bakeries. Nowadays, it seems coffee shops have been strategically placed in every nook and cranny in the airport terminal (not to mention everywhere outside too). If you want some freshly brewed coffee or tea to drink, go for it, but watch out if you want to eat. The muffins (low-fat ones included), scones, pastries, croissants, donuts, and cookies innocently beckoning to you from behind the glass counter are nutritional disasters. They provide an explosion of refined white flour teamed up with sugar (often 6+ teaspoons) that send your blood sugar souring upward, only to crash a bit later. The fallout is hunger and the toxic type of hunger you do not want to develop in the airport or airplane. Please think of these foods as what they really are—powerful appetite stimulants! Of course, it would be an awful idea to begin your day on this grumbling note, so please ignore the verbal prompts for adding a muffin or pastry when you are getting your morning cup of java. If you need breakfast, opt for oatmeal or a veggie and egg wrap if available. Or stick with fresh fruit salad and some yogurt. If you have a hankering for a specialty coffee beverage, keep in mind that many are dripping in excess calories (500 plus) from sugar and saturated fats. Stick to the smallest size and order it light or non-fat, and without the whipped topping.

Jumbo Pretzel Outlets. Back in our misguided, low-fat phase of the eighties and nineties, pretzels somehow garnered a healthy reputation, and it still persists to this day. The scientific reality could not be more counter. A bunch of pure white flour with a bunch of salt (so what if it's low in fat) is definitely not good for you. The blast of glucose and sodium your bloodstream quickly encounters after you eat one of these white flour monstrosities can attack your arteries in many ways and is sure to ring your dinner bell well before it is time for your next meal. If you opt for a sugary versus savory selection, the white flour and salt come along with upwards of seven teaspoons of sugar even before any caramel dipping sauce. Definitely keep your sniffing-distance from this truly twisted food.

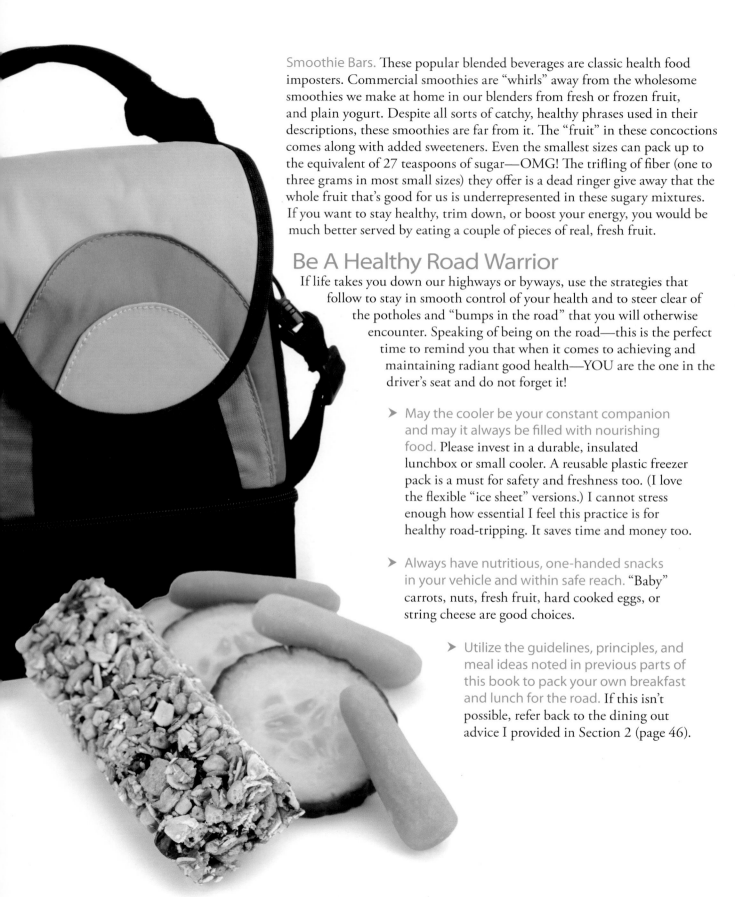

Smoothie Bars. These popular blended beverages are classic health food imposters. Commercial smoothies are "whirls" away from the wholesome smoothies we make at home in our blenders from fresh or frozen fruit, and plain yogurt. Despite all sorts of catchy, healthy phrases used in their descriptions, these smoothies are far from it. The "fruit" in these concoctions comes along with added sweeteners. Even the smallest sizes can pack up to the equivalent of 27 teaspoons of sugar—OMG! The trifling of fiber (one to three grams in most small sizes) they offer is a dead ringer give away that the whole fruit that's good for us is underrepresented in these sugary mixtures. If you want to stay healthy, trim down, or boost your energy, you would be much better served by eating a couple of pieces of real, fresh fruit.

Be A Healthy Road Warrior

If life takes you down our highways or byways, use the strategies that follow to stay in smooth control of your health and to steer clear of the potholes and "bumps in the road" that you will otherwise encounter. Speaking of being on the road—this is the perfect time to remind you that when it comes to achieving and maintaining radiant good health—YOU are the one in the driver's seat and do not forget it!

➤ May the cooler be your constant companion and may it always be filled with nourishing food. Please invest in a durable, insulated lunchbox or small cooler. A reusable plastic freezer pack is a must for safety and freshness too. (I love the flexible "ice sheet" versions.) I cannot stress enough how essential I feel this practice is for healthy road-tripping. It saves time and money too.

➤ Always have nutritious, one-handed snacks in your vehicle and within safe reach. "Baby" carrots, nuts, fresh fruit, hard cooked eggs, or string cheese are good choices.

➤ Utilize the guidelines, principles, and meal ideas noted in previous parts of this book to pack your own breakfast and lunch for the road. If this isn't possible, refer back to the dining out advice I provided in Section 2 (page 46).

If There's A Will...
THERE'S A WAY

I am a big believer in the power of real life stories to teach and empower others and would like to share one of my personal stories with you. In this particular instance, I encountered the single greatest nutritional challenge of all my times on the road. I was visiting the Panhandle of Nebraska for a series of speaking engagements and spent three nights in a very small rural town. My motel did not offer a full service restaurant, but as a courtesy, did provide the menus for the only two dinner dining establishments within a reasonable walking distance. One was a pizzeria and the other a sports bar. I opted for the pizzeria because I spotted from my quick glance at the menu that entrée salads were offered. I walked over, sat in an open booth, and picked up the menu for a closer look. I went right to the salad offerings, but was highly dismayed when I saw that the only vegetables in any of the salads were: iceberg lettuce, romaine lettuce, tomatoes, and pickle spears—talk about veggie anemia!

Already anticipating vegetable withdrawal, my eyes happened upon the list of "available pizza toppings" and bingo! I found what I needed. Included were a bunch of vegetables, even some of my favorite superstars like red onion, broccoli, green bell peppers, red bell peppers, roma tomatoes, black olives, mushrooms, and spinach. I gestured for my waiter and told him that I wanted to order the entrée grilled chicken salad, but with some big changes. He nodded okay and I proceeded. With a voice at once strong, kind, and encouraging, I ordered the following: the grilled chicken salad with romaine lettuce and tomatoes (no iceberg lettuce, croutons or cheese please) topped with a medley of every vegetable topping from the pizza menu (all eight), and the vinaigrette dressing on the side. Because I love the combination of roasted vegetables with fresh, raw veggies in a salad, I made the special request to first roast the veggie toppings in the pizza oven before adding them to the salad. The kitchen staff kindly accommodated all of my wishes, and my dinner salad was absolutely delicious! So delectable, in fact, that I ate it three nights in a row.

The moral of this story: when it comes to healthy eating—if there is a will there will always be a way!

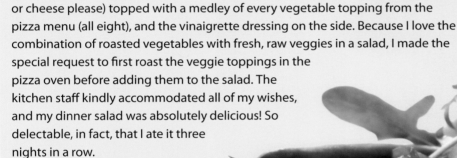

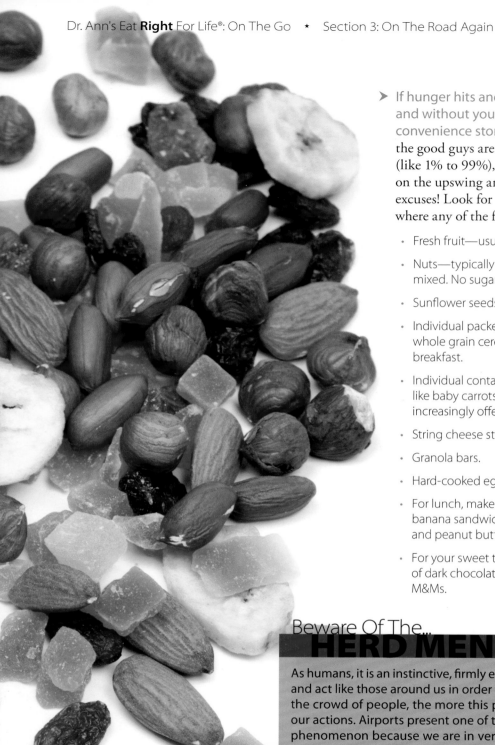

➤ If hunger hits and you find yourself snackless, and without your trusty lunchbox buddy, the convenience store is sure to beckon. Although the good guys are far out-numbered by the bad guys (like 1% to 99%), healthy choices are thankfully on the upswing and can always be found. So no excuses! Look for or simply ask the c-store clerk where any of the following are located:

- Fresh fruit—usually bananas, apples, oranges.

- Nuts—typically almonds, cashews, peanuts or mixed. No sugarcoated versions.

- Sunflower seeds/trail mix.

- Individual packets of plain oatmeal or cold whole grain cereals like plain Cheerios work for breakfast.

- Individual containers of packaged fresh foods like baby carrots, cut up fruit, and yogurt are increasingly offered.

- String cheese sticks.

- Granola bars.

- Hard-cooked eggs.

- For lunch, make your own peanut butter and banana sandwich. 100% whole wheat bread and peanut butter should be on the shelf.

- For your sweet tooth, opt for a prudent portion of dark chocolate or dark chocolate peanut M&Ms.

Beware Of The...
HERD MENTALITY

As humans, it is an instinctive, firmly entrenched behavioral tendency to do and act like those around us in order to feel "part of the crowd." The larger the crowd of people, the more this powerful subliminal force influences our actions. Airports present one of the highest risk environments for this phenomenon because we are in very close proximity to large groups of people. As a frequent traveler who always observes the eating behavior of those around me, I can tell you from vast experience that the longest lines and biggest crowds are at the food outlets that serve up the unhealthiest foods. I encourage you to fight this peer pressure and dare to be different just like I do. There is simply no feeling as empowering and rewarding as being in active control of your own health. Always remember that YOU are the only person that can make YOU healthy and feel proud that you've done the right thing.

Staying Overnight

For the business travelers and road-tripping families (travel soccer or baseball anyone?) that often find themselves bunking up in the budget hotel chains like I do, I have some additional bits of wisdom to help you remain on the highway to health and to stay at the top of your game.

➤ Please just say no to the complimentary cookie at check-in–even if it is freshly baked and warm. This is another pet peeve of mine! Better yet, do what I do and passionately, yet politely request that they aspire to make it easier, not harder for Americans to stay healthy and trim. The fact that they offer these oversized cookies in the age of our unprecedented obesity crisis is simply beyond me.

➤ Be wary of the vending machines you will invariably walk past going to and leaving your room. If you are traveling alone without the watchful eye of others, they may especially tempt you. If you must, hit the button for the nuts, granola bars, sunflower seeds, reduced-fat popcorn, trail mix, dried fruit, whole grain crackers, or baked or multigrain chips, like SunChips.

➤ The free breakfast is convenient and appreciated, but doing it right takes some know-how and attentiveness. I knew I was going to write this book, so I purposely jotted down everything offered at the complimentary breakfast bar during my last three hotel stays. The complete list of offerings included: pastries, white bagels, muffins (all white flour), white bread, dry cereals (Frosted Flakes, Raisin Bran, Fruit Loops), flavored yogurt, scrambled eggs, hard-cooked eggs, sausage, bacon, biscuits and gravy, fresh fruit, and instant oatmeal (plain and flavored). From this list, we have three healthy breakfast meal options.

1. Scrambled or hard-cooked eggs and fresh fruit.

2. Plain oatmeal sweetened with cut up fresh fruit (best to make with 1% or skim milk for extra protein).

3. Whole grain cereal (Raisin Bran) with 1% milk and fresh fruit.

   Really any combination of the above would be fine.

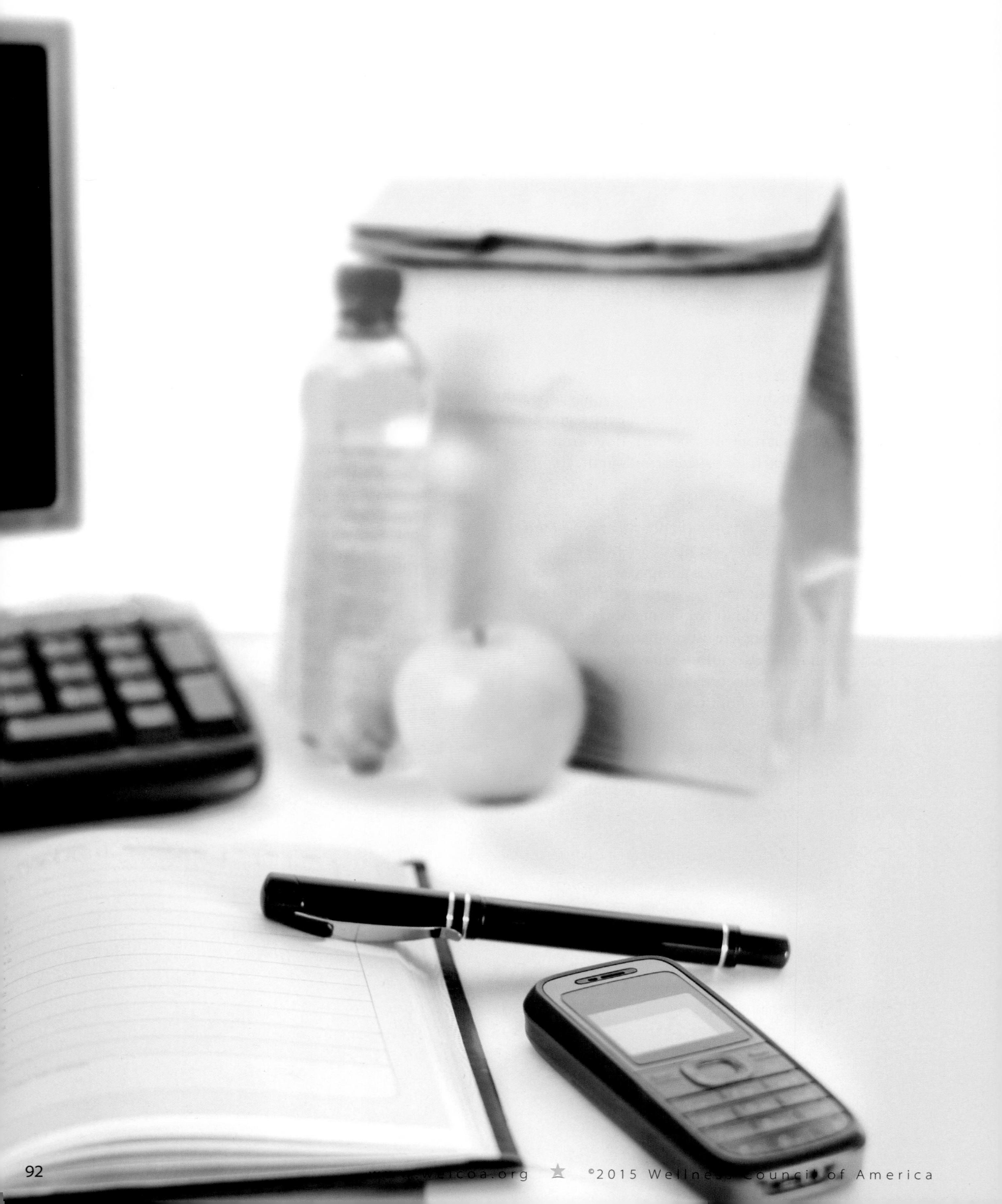

Eating At Work

Eating At Work

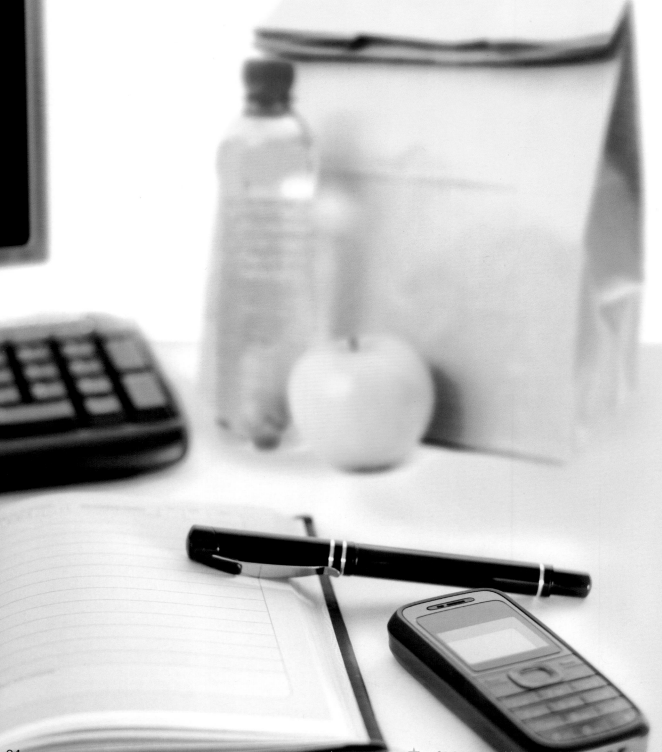

Because our immediate physical surroundings have such an enormous influence on what ultimately enters our mouths, and because most of us spend 40 plus hours a week in the workplace, practicing strict environmental control with your food during the workday is supremely important. I have repeated this many times throughout this book, but I want to remind you again that the Holy Grail for maintaining a healthy diet is ensuring that nutritious foods are readily accessible and unhealthy foods are as inaccessible as possible—in this case, preferably completely off-site or at least out of sight. To maintain your health, your body weight and your work productivity, here are some winning strategies for healthy eating in the workplace.

➤ **Make brown-bagging your lunch (or breakfast) a habit.** When you prepare your own meals you have complete control of their nutritional quality and their portions. The time and money this savvy routine can save you is precious too. Remember also that of all meals, studies show that going out to lunch provides the highest risk for eating too many calories. (To the tune of 159 to 239 extra daily calories.) Over time, this surfeit of lunch calories can really pack on the pounds. Packing a healthy lunch is one of the surest ways to trim your waistline and your budget, while boosting your vim and vigor, so just do it!

➤ **Apply the principles and advice I have shared throughout this book to build the best lunch.** If you want my "cookbook version" of exactly how to make a quick, easy, tasty, healthy and portable lunch for work—I included eight of my favorite lunch recipes in the *Eat Right for Life®: Cookbook Companion.*

➤ **To keep things really efficient and to save you tons of time—let your dinner leftovers double for lunch the next day.** This is always my first choice for workday lunches. For me, the prospect of getting two or more meals from one is a huge motivator for dishing up a healthy dinner generous enough to provide ready-made lunches!

➤ **For snack attacks and the inevitable "no time to pack a lunch" days, take advantage of the office kitchenette.** Stock the refrigerator and cupboards exclusively with good-for-you foods, especially those that are quick and convenient like fresh fruit, finger-friendly cut fresh vegetables, individual containers of hummus and peanut butter, plain yogurt, boiled eggs, cheese sticks, canned tuna or salmon with pop-tops, whole grain crackers, nuts and 70% or higher cacao dark chocolate bars (in moderation). Of course, if it's not there it is not an option so keep the junk foods out of your work environment! The office microwave is great for heating dinner leftovers and other quick lunches like a can of chili, a wholesome can of soup made with beans or vegetables, any variety of rinsed, canned beans paired with diced canned tomatoes, or a "healthy" frozen meal. I am not a fan of frozen meals, but if you must, I think the Kashi and South Beach Diet brands have the best overall nutritional quality.

Germs, Germs EVERYWHERE

When it comes to germs and the average office desk—they are filthy as crap—literally. An eye-opening 2007 laboratory study conducted by University of Arizona researchers found that the average office work desk harbors 400 times more bacteria than a toilet seat—Yuck!

Other particularly germy office spots were phones, microwave door handles, water fountain handles (another reason to bring your own water bottle) and keyboards. Thankfully, a follow-up investigation by the same researchers found that simply wiping down the desk area once a day with disinfecting wipes reduced germ levels by 99.9 percent. So keep those wipes handy and use them!

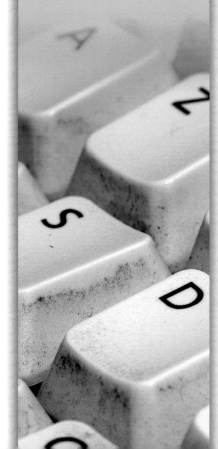

> Be mindful of food safety issues. Always wash your hands before eating with plain soap and water. Hand sanitizers are not a replacement for hand washing. Simply washing your hands remains one of the most effective means of reducing your risk of getting infections, including food-borne illness. According to the experts, rubbing your hands together with soap (no antibacterial soap required) under running water for 20 seconds, rinsing them in clean water, and then drying them with a clean towel or air-drying them is best. Be sure your office microwave and refrigerator—especially their handles—are regularly cleaned. If they are not, they will become a petri dish for bacterial growth.

> Choose your dining partners wisely. Social influences have a demonstrable impact on what and how much we eat. Because we naturally want to fit in, we tend to do as those with us do. Based on one recent study, it seems we "mirror" the overall eating behavior of those we are dining with, especially in the initial part of the meal. Scientists believe it is an intrinsic behavioral tendency to adjust what we eat—whether it be more or less—based on what our dining companions do. I encourage you to seek the company of others to share your mealtime with because eating in solitude can be lonely and also increases the risk of over consumption. However, be attentive in choosing the companionship of healthy eaters. This will make nutritional success easier for you. Assuming that healthy eating and healthy friendships are your goals, NEVER be openly judgmental of other's eating habits, but always be proud to proclaim that you are determined to take full advantage of the remarkable power of the right foods to boost your health, happiness, and work productivity. Take it from me as someone who never misses the opportunity to plug and model healthy eating—your example can be very influential!

Practice Leftover...
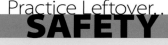
SAFETY

> Package any leftovers in sealed, airtight containers to a depth of no more than two inches to speed chilling. I recommend microwave-safe glass or ceramic containers over plastic containers due to potentially unhealthy compounds that may leach from the plastic into your food.

> Put all leftovers in the refrigerator within two hours of cooking.

> Consume any cooked leftovers within four days.

> Preheat leftovers to a temperature of 165° F before eating them.

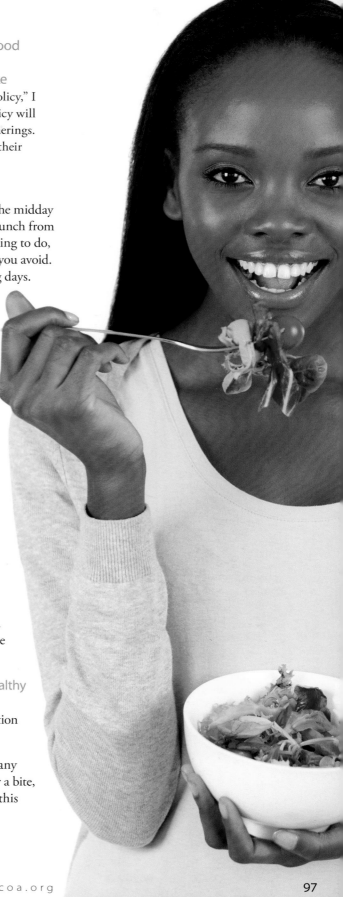

➤ For office lunches or other work-related gatherings where food is being served, use the principles I have equipped you with throughout our *Eat Right For Life®: On The Go* journey to make smart choices. If your workplace does not have a "healthy food policy," I encourage you to take the lead and push for one. The best food policy will cover the company cafeteria, the vending machines, and office gatherings. WELCOA has samples of model food policies as free resources on their website **www.welcoa.org**.

Desk-Dining Do's

Although I highly recommend that you take your lunch elsewhere for the midday respite you deserve, I know that many of you will nonetheless eat your lunch from your desk or work station. On the surface, it may seem like a sensible thing to do, but it comes with several not-so-obvious drawbacks that I want to help you avoid. Use the tips that follow to take the dicey out of your desk-bound dining days.

➤ First and foremost, do stay mindful of your meal. Take your mind off of work and put it all into your mouth and onto your plate. Forget the phone, the internet and the emails. Eating mindlessly, especially in front of distracting influences like your computer, invites overconsumption. Overeating is one of the biggest dangers of desktop dining so be forewarned!

➤ If you decide to eat at your desk, do make a concerted effort to stand up and move more often during other parts of the day. Sitting for eight hours a day is bad enough and desk-dining can push it to nine—ouch that really hurts!

➤ Do keep the food on your plate and your hands away from the mouse, keyboard, and phone as you eat. Any crumbs or food residues that spill over onto your desk or things you may touch with foodie fingers will become a fertile breeding ground for bacteria. Placemats can add a bit of civility to your meal and protect your desk from food contamination.

➤ Do sanitize your desk regularly. Wiping your desk area down with disinfecting wipes at the start of each day is a very wise habit. Be especially diligent in de-germing high hand traffic areas like the mouse, keyboard, and phone handset.

➤ Do invite a colleague to join you (preferably one who has a healthy meal, too). The social interaction is good for your heart and soul, improves workplace relationships, and provides a welcome distraction from work-related worries.

➤ Do keep a spill-proof water bottle on your desk at all times. Many times we mistake thirst for hunger. Before you reach for a snack or a bite, take a long tall sip of water first. You may find like I often do that this zero calorie oral stimulation hits the spot just fine.

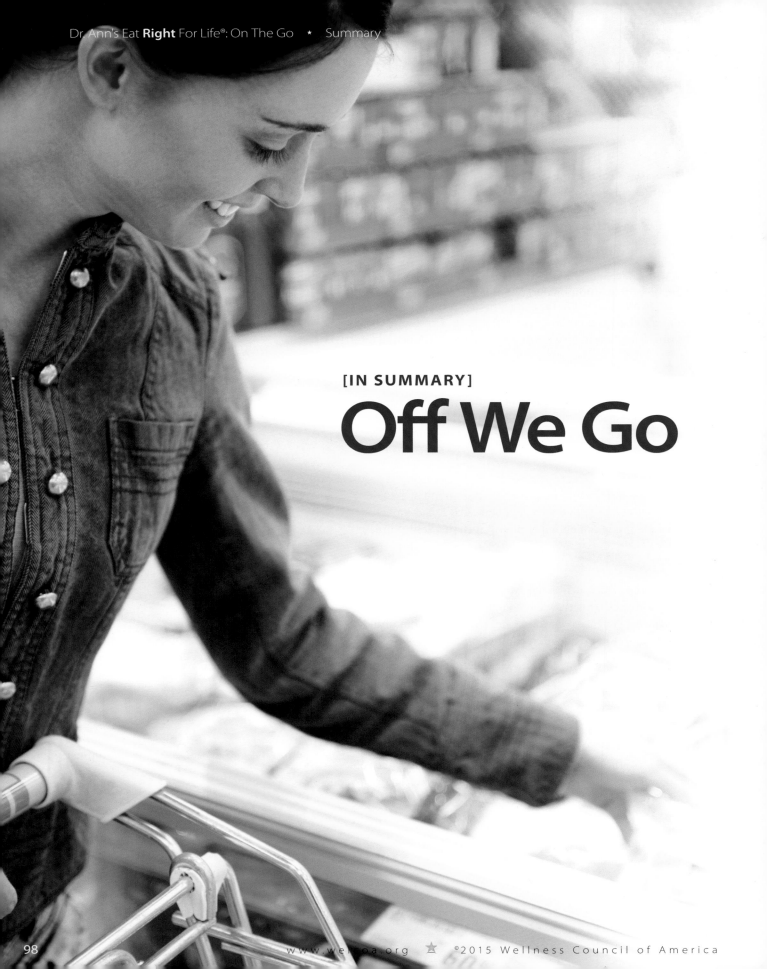

[IN SUMMARY]

Off We Go

I want to thank you for the pleasure of allowing me to share my *"Eat Right For Life®: On The Go"* guidance with you. Regardless of where life may take you into our formidable food culture, I have complete confidence that you can have resounding nutritional success with the information that I have shared in this book. Despite how busy and hectic life can be—I know that you have the power to select foods and meals that nourish and sustain your health without compromising the joys, ease, and convenience of eating in the real world. All it takes is a little wisdom and determination, and I promise you that the energy and vitality you get in return will be a reward to relish forever. Optimal health is an infinitely gratifying, yet easily attainable achievement, and you owe it to yourself and your family to get there.

As you venture out into your external food environment with your new found nutritional insight and take-charge-of-your-plate attitude, I would be delighted to hear from you and welcome your feedback at www.DrAnnWellness.com. If you are hungry for additional knowledge and inspiration, I have a full library of free wellness resources available from my website, and I encourage you to take full advantage of them. I am determined to help you live your healthiest life and have created my video tips, monthly e-newsletter, blog, and a host of other helpful resources just for you. If you want to get really personal and receive a daily dose of my wellness wisdom, jump on board with me at Twitter (@DrAnnWellness) and Facebook.

Lastly, I would like to thank my good friends at The Wellness Council of America (WELCOA) for bringing my words to life with this visually stunning and irresistibly engaging book. Words are inadequate to convey the depth and breadth of gratitude I feel for our partnership and the extraordinary work and enthusiastic devotion they commit to improving the health and well-being of working Americans.

On behalf of both of us, I am speaking straight from the heart when I say, we wish you the very best of health and will always be cheering you on in your wellness endeavors.

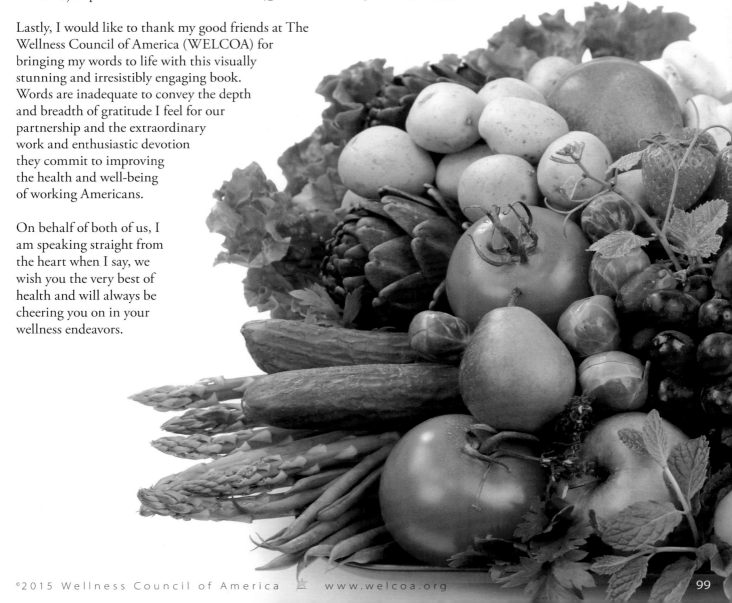

Citations

Morbidity and Mortality Weekly Report Centers for Disease Control and Nutritional Institutes of Health 60:41, 2011

The American Journal of Clinical Nutrition 85:1, 2007

The American Journal of Clinical Nutrition 91:2, 2010

Lancet 365:9471, 2005

Archives of Pediatrics and Adolescent Medicine 159:7, 2005

The American Journal of Clinical Nutrition 83:2, 2006

How Food Away From Home Affects Children's Diet Quality. ERR – 104. U.S. Department of Agriculture, Economic Research Service October 2010

The American Journal of Clinical Nutrition 88:5, 2008

American College of Nutrition 23:2, 2004

Critical Public Health 21:4, 2011

Proceedings of the National Academy Sciences 105:46, 2008

American Journal of Epidemiology 168:12, 2008

Journal of Alzheimer's Disease 16:1, 2009

The Impact of Food Away From Home On Adult Diet Quality. ERR – 90 USDA, Economic Research Service February 2010

Food Policy 34:6, 2010

The American Journal of Clinical Nutrition 6:85, 2007

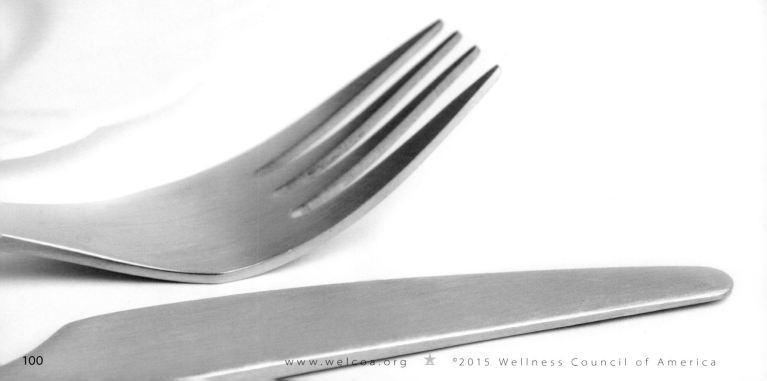